The pregnancy Diet And Cookbook

Nourishing Recipes and Meal Plans for a Healthy Pregnancy

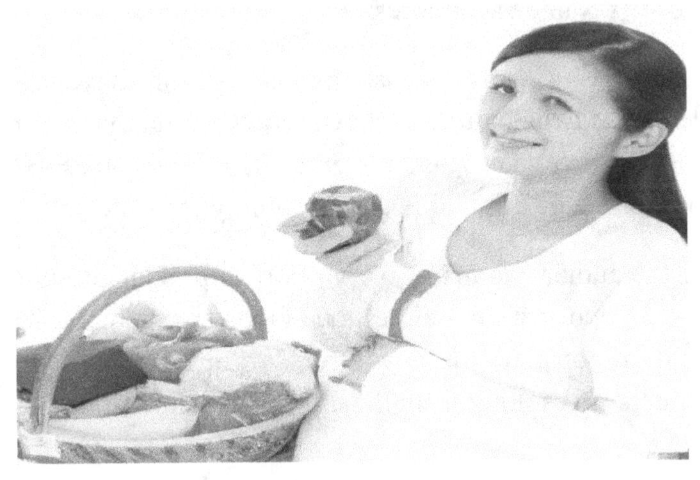

Dr. Mary K. Clubb

Copyright © [2023] by [Dr. Mary K. Clubb]

This book is a work of non-fiction. All of the characters, incidents, and dialogue are drawn from the author's personal experiences, interviews, and research. Any resemblance to actual persons, living or dead, or events is entirely coincidental.

While the author has made every effort to provide accurate and up-to-date information, neither the author nor the publisher can be held responsible for any errors or omissions or for any consequences resulting from the use of this information.

Table of Contents

1.0 Introduction to the Pregnancy Diet

Gloria was happy to find that she was pregnant. She and her husband had been hoping for a baby for a while, and now that it had finally occurred, she wanted to do everything she could to guarantee a successful pregnancy.

One of the things Gloria was most worried about was her nutrition. She understood that consuming the correct meals throughout pregnancy was vital for her and her kid's health. Yet Gloria was a gourmet at heart, and the notion of giving up her favourite meals for nine months was overwhelming.

Eager to make the most of her pregnant diet, Gloria hit the books and began studying healthful meals. She uncovered much information on diet and pregnancy and found a recipe suited to pregnant women.
Equipped with her new knowledge, Gloria started to work in the kitchen. She experimented with various ingredients and developed tasty, healthful meals that fulfilled her desires and nutritional demands. She made careful to incorporate enough leafy greens, lean meats, and whole grains in her diet, as well as healthy fats and a variety of fruits and vegetables.

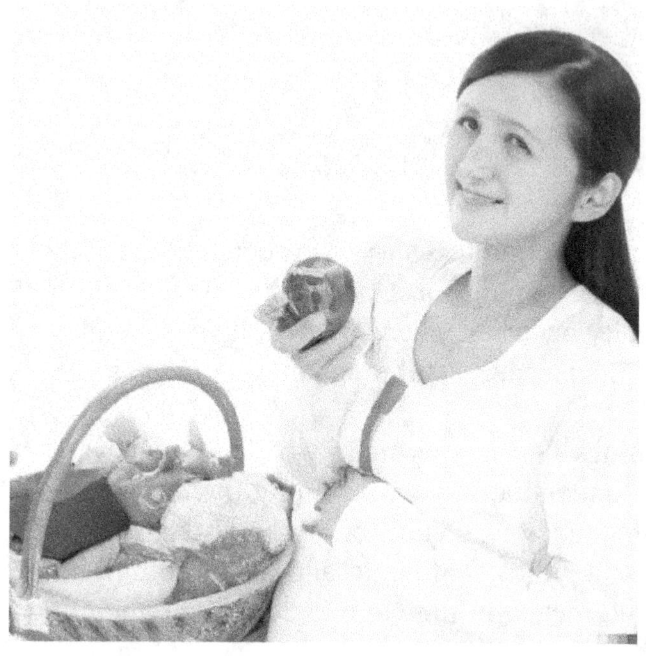

As her pregnancy proceeded, Gloria started to feel more and more secure in her abilities to nurture herself and her developing baby. She liked trying new foods and even began sharing them with her friends and family.

Gloria's pregnancy diet became a routine as the months went by. She started to enjoy planning and preparing nutritious meals and found that it gave her a sense of purpose and fulfilment. She even started to get creative with her cooking, experimenting with different herbs and spices to add flavour to her dishes.

One of the things that Gloria loved most about her pregnancy diet was how it made her feel. She had more energy and felt healthier overall. She also noticed that her mood was more stable and had fewer pregnancy-related symptoms like nausea and fatigue.

As her due date approached, Gloria made sure to stock up on healthy snacks and easy-to-prepare meals for the postpartum period. She knew she would need plenty of nourishing foods to support her body as it healed and recovered from childbirth.

When the day finally came to meet her little one, Gloria felt proud of the effort she had put into her pregnancy diet. She knew she had done everything possible to give her baby the best possible start. As she held her newborn in her arms, Gloria felt deep gratitude and joy, knowing she had played a vital role in bringing this precious new life into the world.

When her baby finally arrived, Gloria was grateful for the support and encouragement of her healthcare providers, who had emphasized the importance of a healthy pregnancy diet throughout her pregnancy. She felt confident in her ability to continue making healthy food choices as she embarked on motherhood.

Looking back on her pregnancy, Gloria was grateful for the experience of exploring new foods and learning more about nutrition. She knew that the habits she had formed during pregnancy would serve her well for years and that she had set a healthy example for her growing family.

A healthy diet is crucial during pregnancy, as it provides the essential nutrients needed to support the growth and development of the growing baby. Eating correctly throughout pregnancy may also assist in lowering the risk of difficulties and ensure a healthy pregnancy.

The Prenatal Diet Cookbook is a complete guide to healthy eating throughout pregnancy, aimed to assist pregnant women in making educated decisions about their nutrition. Whether you're a seasoned cook or a beginner in the kitchen, this cookbook provides practical advice and delicious recipes to help you eat well throughout your pregnancy.

In the first Chapter, we'll explore the nutritional requirements during pregnancy, including the recommended daily intake of calories, protein, carbohydrates, fats, and essential vitamins and minerals. We'll also discuss how to plan and prepare nutritious meals, including healthy snack options for busy days.
Subsequent chapters will be dedicated to breakfast, lunch, dinner, snacks, desserts, drinks, and smoothies, focusing on delicious, nutrient-rich recipes that are easy to prepare and satisfying to eat.

We'll also provide tips for managing pregnancy-related conditions, such as gestational diabetes and preeclampsia, with dietary recommendations and tailored recipes.

At the end of each Chapter, you'll find a summary of the essential nutritional information, along with practical tips and advice to help you make the most of your pregnancy diet. Following this cookbook's guidance, you can enjoy a healthy, balanced diet that supports your and your baby's health.

We hope this cookbook will be a valuable resource for expecting mothers everywhere, empowering you to make informed choices about your diet and enjoy a happy, healthy pregnancy.

1.1 Why a healthy diet is essential during pregnancy

A healthy diet is vital during pregnancy because it provides nutrients for the mother and the growing baby. Pregnancy is a time of significant physical and hormonal changes, which can add stress to the body.
Eating a balanced and nutritious diet can help to support the mother's health and well-being, as well as the health of the developing fetus.

Here are some of the key reasons why a healthy diet is essential during pregnancy:

Supports fetal development: The nutrients from the mother's diet are the building blocks for the baby's growth and development. A diet rich in essential vitamins, minerals, and macronutrients like protein and carbohydrates can help to support the development of the baby's brain, organs, and tissues.
Reduces the risk of complications: Eating a healthy diet during pregnancy can help to reduce the risk of

complications like gestational diabetes, preeclampsia, and preterm birth. Adequate nutrition can also help to prevent low birth weight and other adverse pregnancy outcomes.

Provides energy: Pregnancy can be physically demanding, and a healthy diet can help to provide the energy needed to support the mother's daily activities and the baby's growth.

Boosts the immune system: A healthy diet can help to support the immune system, which is essential during pregnancy as the mother's body is more susceptible to infections.

Improves mood: The hormonal changes during pregnancy can lead to mood swings and other emotional challenges. Eating a healthy diet can help to improve mood and reduce stress.

Helps with postpartum recovery: A healthy diet can also help to support postpartum recovery as the mother's body heals and recovers from childbirth.

A healthy diet is essential for both the mother and the developing baby during pregnancy. It is vital to prioritize nutrient-dense foods like fruits, vegetables, lean proteins, whole grains, and healthy fats and to limit processed and high-fat foods. A balanced and varied diet can help support the mother's health and well-being, well-being, and the growing baby's healthy growth and development.

Eating a healthy and balanced diet during pregnancy is crucial for supporting the growth and development of the growing fetus. A mother's diet provides the essential nutrients that the fetus needs for proper development, which can lead to complications and adverse outcomes.

Here are some of the critical nutrients that are important for fetal development:

Folic acid: Folic acid is a B vitamin essential for proper fetal brain and spinal cord development. Adequate folic acid intake during pregnancy can help to prevent congenital disabilities like spina bifida.

Iron is essential for forming red blood cells and transporting oxygen to the fetus. Iron deficiency during pregnancy can lead to anaemia and low birth weight.

Calcium: Calcium is essential for developing the baby's bones and teeth. A lack of calcium during pregnancy can lead to bone density loss in the mother and the baby.

Protein: Protein is necessary for developing the baby's tissues, muscles, and organs.

Omega-3 fatty acids: Omega-3 fatty acids, found in fatty fish and other sources, are essential for developing the baby's brain and eyes.

Vitamin D: Vitamin D is essential for the absorption of calcium and the development of the baby's bones and teeth.

It's important to note that a healthy and balanced diet can provide these nutrients in the appropriate amounts. However, some women may require supplementation if they cannot meet their nutrient needs through diet alone. It's always best to consult a healthcare provider before taking any supplements during pregnancy.

Overall, a healthy and balanced diet during pregnancy is crucial for supporting the growth and development of the fetus. By prioritizing nutrient-dense foods and eating a varied and balanced diet, expecting mothers can help to provide the essential nutrients needed for a healthy pregnancy and a healthy baby.

1.1.2 Reduces the risk of complications

Eating a healthy and balanced diet during pregnancy can help reduce the risk of complications arising during pregnancy and childbirth. Adequate nutrition can help to support the mother's health and well-being, as well as the healthy growth and development of the fetus.

Here are some of the critical complications that can be prevented or reduced with a healthy diet:

Gestational diabetes: Gestational diabetes is a type of diabetes that develops during pregnancy. Eating a healthy and balanced diet can help to regulate blood sugar levels and reduce the risk of gestational diabetes.

Preeclampsia is a severe pregnancy complication with high blood pressure and organ damage. Eating a healthy diet and maintaining a healthy weight can help to reduce the risk of preeclampsia.

Preterm birth: Preterm birth, or birth before 37 weeks of pregnancy, can lead to complications and health issues for the baby. Adequate nutrition can help to reduce the risk of preterm birth.

Low birth weight: Inadequate nutrition during pregnancy can lead to low birth weight, which can increase the risk of health problems for the baby.

Neural tube problems: Neural tube defects are congenital abnormalities that affect the brain and spinal cord. Sufficient folic acid consumption, which may be gained via a healthy dict or supplementation, can assist in avoiding neural tube abnormalities.

It's crucial to remember that although a good diet may assist in lowering the risk of problems, additional variables might contribute to these difficulties, like genetics and pre-existing medical issues. Contacting a healthcare expert for specialized guidance and treatment throughout pregnancy is always better.

Maintaining a nutritious and balanced diet throughout pregnancy may assist in lowering the risk of problems and ensure a successful pregnancy and delivery result. By selecting nutrient-dense diets and avoiding harmful foods, expecting moms may assist in promoting their health and the health of their developing baby.

1.1.3 Gives energy

Pregnancy may be physically taxing, and a good diet is crucial for supplying the energy required to maintain the mother's changing body and the developing baby. A balanced and nutrient-dense diet may assist in ensuring that the mother is receiving the fuel needed to keep up with the demands of pregnancy.

These are some of the significant nutrients that are necessary for giving energy throughout pregnancy:

Carbohydrates: Carbohydrates are the primary energy source for the body, and they offer glucose, which is essential for brain function and physical activity. Complex carbs, like whole grains and vegetables, are the most excellent option for sustained energy throughout the day.

Protein: Protein is vital for creating and repairing tissues, as well as for generating energy. Sufficient protein consumption may assist in avoiding muscle loss and support healthy weight growth during pregnancy.

Iron is essential for developing red blood cells, which deliver oxygen to the body's tissues. Anaemia, which may be caused by iron deficiency, can lead to weariness and reduced energy levels.

B-vitamins: B-vitamins, such as thiamin, riboflavin, and niacin, are required for turning food into energy. A deficit in these vitamins may lead to weariness and lowered energy levels.

Hydration: Keeping hydrated is vital for sustaining energy levels throughout pregnancy. Dehydration may lead to weariness and impaired physical and mental performance.

It's vital to remember that although a nutritious diet may supply the energy required throughout pregnancy, it's also necessary to relax and prevent overexertion. Pregnancy is a time to heed your body's signals and pause when needed.

Overall, eating a balanced and nutrient-dense diet throughout pregnancy may assist in supplying the energy required to meet the demands of pregnancy. Expecting moms may help maintain energy levels and encourage a healthy and active pregnancy by emphasizing complex carbs, protein, and water.

1.1.4 Boosts the immune system

A balanced diet during pregnancy may assist in maintaining the immune system and lower the risk of infections and diseases that can affect the mother and the growing baby. A healthy immune system is essential during pregnancy since the body's immune system is usually reduced to prevent the mother's body from rejecting the growing child.

These are some of the primary nutrients that may aid in boosting the immune system during pregnancy:
Vitamin C: Vitamin C is an antioxidant that helps to protect the body's cells from harm and may aid in strengthening the immune system. Citrus fruits, strawberries, and kiwi are all rich sources of vitamin C.

Vitamin E: Vitamin E is an antioxidant that may aid in strengthening the immune system by protecting cells from harm. Nuts, seeds, and vegetable oils are all rich sources of vitamin E.

Zinc: Zinc is vital for forming immune cells and may assist in avoiding infections. Excellent sources of zinc include meat, poultry, shellfish, beans, and nuts.

Probiotics: Probiotics are "good" bacteria that may aid in strengthening the immune system by supporting a healthy gut microbiome. Yoghurt, kefir, and fermented veggies are all rich sources of probiotics.

Hydration: Keeping hydrated is also vital for boosting the immune system. Water and herbal teas may assist in keeping the body hydrated and promote the body's natural detoxification processes.

It's essential to remember that although a nutritious diet may assist in improving the immune system, other factors can also contribute to a compromised immune system, such as stress and lack of sleep. Contacting a healthcare expert for specialized guidance and treatment throughout pregnancy is always better.

Overall, eating a balanced and nutrient-dense diet throughout pregnancy may improve the immune system and promote the health of the mother and the growing baby. By emphasizing foods high in vitamin C, vitamin E, zinc, and probiotics and keeping hydrated, expecting women may assist in building a healthy and robust immune system throughout pregnancy.

1.1.5 Improves mood

A nutritious diet during pregnancy may also enhance mood and minimize the risk of mood disorders, such as sadness and anxiety. Pregnancy may be an emotional period, and it's crucial to encourage mental and emotional health alongside physical health.
These are some of the primary nutrients that might aid in increasing mood during pregnancy:

Omega-3 fatty acids: Omega-3 fatty acids, especially EPA and DHA, are vital for brain function and may help to lessen the risk of depression and anxiety. Excellent sources of omega-3 fatty acids include fatty fish, such as salmon and tuna, as well as walnuts and flaxseeds.

B-vitamins: B-vitamins, such as folate, B6, and B12, are necessary for brain function and may help to lessen the risk of depression and anxiety. Excellent sources of B vitamins include whole grains, leafy greens, and animal products, such as meat and eggs.

Vitamin D: Vitamin D is vital for mood regulation, and a deficit in vitamin D has been related to an increased risk of depression. Sun exposure and fortified foods, such as milk and orange juice, are excellent sources of vitamin D.

Magnesium: Magnesium is vital for nerve function and may assist in alleviating tension and anxiety. Excellent sources of magnesium include leafy greens, almonds, and whole grains.

Hydration: Keeping hydrated is also vital for mood management. Dehydration may lead to weariness and irritation, contributing to a poor mood.

It's important to note that while a healthy diet can help improve mood, it's also essential to seek professional support if experiencing persistent depression or anxiety during pregnancy.

Overall, eating a balanced and nutrient-dense diet during pregnancy can help to improve mood and support mental and emotional health. By prioritizing foods rich in omega-3 fatty acids, B vitamins, vitamin D, and magnesium and staying hydrated, expecting mothers can help to promote a positive mood and overall well-being during pregnancy.

A healthy diet during pregnancy can also help with postpartum recovery, as it can support healing and provide energy for the demands of breastfeeding and caring for a newborn.

Here are some of the critical nutrients that can help with postpartum recovery:

Protein: Protein is essential for tissue repair and can help to support postpartum healing. Good protein sources include lean meats, poultry, fish, eggs, beans, and tofu.

Iron: Iron is essential for oxygen transport and can help to prevent postpartum anaemia. Good sources of iron include red meat, poultry, fish, beans, and fortified cereals.

Calcium: Calcium is essential for bone health and can help to prevent postpartum osteoporosis. Good sources of calcium include dairy products, leafy greens, and fortified foods, such as orange juice and tofu.

Fibre: Fiber is essential for digestive health and can help to prevent constipation, which is common postpartum. Good sources of fibre include fruits, vegetables, whole grains, and beans.

Hydration: Keeping hydrated is also vital for postpartum healing. Consuming adequate water may assist to boost milk production and avoid dehydration.

It's crucial to remember that postpartum healing may differ from person to person, and it's vital to listen to the body's particular requirements and seek expert care if enduring prolonged pain or difficulties.

Overall, eating a balanced and nutrient-dense diet throughout pregnancy may aid in boosting postpartum recovery by supplying vital nutrients for healing and energy. By emphasizing meals rich in protein, iron, calcium, and fibre and keeping hydrated, pregnant women may assist in ensuring a good recovery after delivery.

Maria had just given birth to her first child and felt overwhelmed by parenting obligations. She battled with postpartum recovery and felt exhausted from the long nights and regular feedings.

Her buddy advised that she concentrate on her food to aid her recovery, so Maria made some adjustments. She started incorporating more protein into her meals by adding chicken and tofu. She included plenty of leafy greens and fortified foods to get enough calcium and iron.

Maria also tried to drink more water throughout the day, which helped her stay hydrated and support her milk production. She even started meal prepping on the weekends, so she always had healthy snacks and meals ready.

As time passed, Maria began noticing a difference in her energy levels and overall well-being. She felt more robust and more capable of handling the demands of parenting, and she was glad for the support of a balanced diet in her postpartum recovery.

During her experience, Maria learnt the significance of prioritizing her health and well-being, particularly during a challenging period like postpartum recovery. She also knew that modest improvements to her nutrition and self-care regimen might significantly impact her physical and mental well-being.

1.2 What to anticipate from the book

The Prenatal Diet Cookbook is a complete handbook for expecting women who wish to focus on their health and well-being throughout pregnancy. Here's what you can anticipate from the book:

Nutrient-rich dishes: The book offers over 100 tasty and nutrient-dense recipes for pregnant women. Each dish contains thorough nutrition information to help pregnant women make educated meal decisions.

Advice on necessary nutrients: The book gives in-depth information on vital nutrients for a healthy pregnancy, including protein, iron, calcium, and omega-3 fatty acids. It also includes recommendations on integrating these nutrients into meals and snacks throughout the day.

Suggestions for managing common pregnant symptoms: The book contains tips on handling typical pregnancy symptoms, such as nausea, exhaustion, and constipation. It also includes ideas for items that might help ease these symptoms.

Meal planning and preparation tips: The book contains instructions on planning and preparing meals and snacks for a healthy pregnancy. It suggests meal preparation, grocery shopping, and bulk cooking to make healthy eating more practical for pregnant women.

Information on food safety: The book contains information on food safety during pregnancy, including instructions on preventing foodborne diseases and guidelines for proper food handling and preparation.

Techniques for postpartum recovery: The book provides information on how to assist postpartum recovery via diet, with advice on consuming nutrient-rich meals that may help in healing and give energy for the demands of nursing and caring for a baby.

Overall, The Prenatal Diet Cookbook is a fantastic resource for expecting women who wish to emphasize their health and the health of their developing kid. It gives practical counsel, delectable recipes, and critical nutrition and postpartum recovery information, making it an invaluable tool for a healthy and enjoyable pregnant journey.

2.0 Nutritional Needs during Pregnancy

2.1 Suggested daily consumption of calories, protein, carbs, and lipids

The recommended daily consumption of calories, protein, carbs, and lipids during pregnancy varies based on a woman's specific requirements and stage of pregnancy. Nonetheless, the following are broad guidelines:

Calories: Pregnant women need 300-500 calories daily to promote fetal growth and development. This puts the total recommended daily consumption at 2,200-2,900 calories for most women.

Protein: Protein is needed for the growth and development of fetal tissues and for maternal tissue growth and repair. The recommended daily intake of protein during pregnancy is 75-100 grams per day. Excellent sources of protein include lean meats, fish, poultry, beans, nuts, and dairy products.

Carbohydrates: Carbohydrates are vital for the mother and the growing fetus. Carbs are recommended during pregnancy, and consume 175-210 grams daily. Healthy sources of carbs include fruits, vegetables, whole grains, and legumes.

Fats: Fats are essential for the development of the embryonic brain and nervous system, as well as for the absorption of fat-soluble vitamins. The recommended daily intake of fats during pregnancy is 20-35% of total daily calories. Excellent sources of healthful fats include avocados, nuts, seeds, fatty seafood, and olive oil.

It's crucial for pregnant women to engage with their healthcare practitioner to identify their particular nutritional requirements and to ensure they are achieving their recommended daily intake of calories, protein, carbs, and fats. A nutritious and balanced diet during pregnancy may assist in promoting fetal growth and development, lower the risk of problems, and enhance the mother's well-being.

2.2 Necessary vitamins and minerals during pregnancy

Women must take various necessary vitamins and minerals throughout pregnancy to promote fetal growth, development, and maternal health. Some of the most critical vitamins and minerals during pregnancy include:

Folic Acid: Folic acid is necessary for the formation of the neural tube, which produces the baby's brain and spinal cord. Pregnant women should ingest at least 600-800 mcg of folic acid every day. Excellent sources of folic acid include leafy green vegetables, beans, and fortified cereals.

Iron: Iron is essential for developing red blood cells, which supply oxygen to the infant. Pregnant women should strive to ingest 27 mg of iron each day. Excellent sources of iron include lean red meat, chicken, fish, beans, and fortified grains.

Calcium: Calcium is vital for developing the baby's bones and teeth. Pregnant women should strive to ingest 1,000-1,300 mg of calcium daily. Excellent sources of calcium include milk, cheese, yoghurt, tofu, and leafy green vegetables.

Vitamin D: Vitamin D is vital for the absorption of calcium and the development of the baby's bones and teeth. Pregnant women should attempt to ingest 600-800 international units (IU) of vitamin D per day. Excellent sources of vitamin D include fortified milk, fatty salmon, and exposure to sunshine.

Omega-3 Fatty Acids: Omega-3 fatty acids are vital for developing the baby's brain and eyes. Pregnant women should strive to take 200-300 mg of omega-3 fatty acids each day. Excellent sources of omega-3 fatty acids include fatty fish, flaxseed, and chia seeds.

In addition to these vital vitamins and minerals, pregnant women should also ensure they are ingesting enough levels of other nutrients, such as vitamin C, vitamin A, and zinc. A balanced and varied diet that includes a range of nutrient-dense foods will assist in guaranteeing pregnant women, and their growing kids obtain the nutrients they need for optimum health.

Folic acid, often known as folate, is a B vitamin that plays a vital role in the development of a healthy fetus. It is especially critical during the early stages of pregnancy when the neural tube is developing. Neural tube abnormalities may develop when the neural tube fails to shut correctly, leading to significant birth problems.

Pregnant women are urged to ingest at least 600-800 mcg of folic acid daily. This may be done with a balanced diet that includes leafy green vegetables, beans, citrus fruits, and fortified cereals. In addition, several prenatal vitamins also contain folic acid to ensure pregnant women are fulfilling their daily needs.
It's vital for women to start ingesting proper levels of folic acid before pregnancy since the neural tube begins to grow only 3-4 weeks after conception - frequently before a woman even realizes she's pregnant. Thus, it's suggested that women of reproductive age ingest 400 micrograms of folic acid daily, even if they're not actively attempting to conceive.

Although folic acid is crucial during pregnancy, it's also essential for general health. Folic acid is involved in the formation of red blood cells and helps avoid anaemia. It's also been related to a lower risk of heart disease and stroke.

Pregnant women must chat with their healthcare practitioner about their folic acid consumption and ensure they fulfil their daily needs for a safe pregnancy.

2.2.2 Iron

Iron is vital in developing red blood cells, transporting oxygen throughout the body. Throughout pregnancy, a woman's blood volume rises to support the growing baby, which increases her iron demands.

Pregnant women are suggested to ingest 27 mg of iron per day, which may be gained via a nutritious diet that includes red meat, chicken, fish, beans, and fortified cereals. In addition, several prenatal vitamins now include iron to ensure pregnant women are reaching their daily needs.

Iron deficiency is frequent during pregnancy and may lead to anaemia, a disease in which the body doesn't have enough red blood cells. Anaemia may induce weariness, weakness, and a diminished capacity to fight infections. Severe iron deficiency during pregnancy may significantly raise the risk of preterm delivery and low birth weight.

It's crucial for pregnant women to consult with their healthcare practitioner about their iron consumption and ensure they're fulfilling their daily needs for a safe pregnancy. In rare circumstances, a healthcare physician may offer an iron supplement to avoid iron deficiency anaemia.

It's also crucial to remember that ingesting meals high in vitamin C may enhance iron absorption from plant-based sources. For example, mixing a spinach salad with a citrus fruit will assist in boosting iron absorption.

2.2.3 Calcium

Calcium is a mineral that is vital for forming healthy bones and teeth. During pregnancy, a woman's body requires extra calcium to promote the baby's skeleton's growth and maintain her bone density.
Pregnant women are suggested to ingest 1,000-1,300 mg of calcium per day, which may be gained via a balanced diet that includes dairy products, leafy green vegetables, tofu, and fortified foods. In addition, several prenatal vitamins also include calcium to ensure pregnant women are fulfilling their daily needs.

Calcium is also crucial for muscle and neuron function, blood coagulation, and the release of hormones. If a pregnant woman doesn't ingest enough calcium, her body will remove the calcium it needs from her bones, which may lead to lower bone density and an increased risk of osteoporosis later in life.

Pregnant women must discuss with their healthcare practitioner about their calcium consumption and ensure they're achieving their daily needs for a safe pregnancy. A healthcare physician may suggest a calcium supplement to fulfil daily needs in rare circumstances.

It's also vital to know that taking adequate vitamin D is required for the body to absorb and utilize calcium. Excellent dietary sources of vitamin D include fatty fish, egg yolks, and fortified foods. Sun exposure is also a source of vitamin D, although pregnant women should speak to their healthcare professionals about safe sun exposure and the need for a vitamin D supplement.

2.2.4 Vitamin D

Vitamin D is essential for maintaining bone health and boosting the immune system. Vitamin D is especially critical for developing the fetal skeleton during pregnancy since it helps the body absorb calcium and stimulates bone formation.

Vitamin D may be gained from sun exposure since the body creates vitamin D when the skin is exposed to UVB light. Nonetheless, pregnant women should be careful about sun exposure and speak to their healthcare professionals about acceptable amounts of sun exposure and the need for a vitamin D supplement.

Dietary sources of vitamin D include fatty fish such as salmon and tuna, egg yolks, and fortified foods such as milk and orange juice. Yet, receiving sufficient vitamin D from food alone may be challenging, especially during the winter months when sun exposure is restricted.

The recommended daily dosage of vitamin D for pregnant women is 600-800 IU per day, depending on age and other variables. Pregnant women should consult their healthcare practitioner about their vitamin D requirements and whether a supplement is essential to support a safe pregnancy.

2.2.5 Omega-3 Fatty Acids

Omega-3 fatty acids are a form of unsaturated fat crucial for developing the embryonic brain and eyes. During pregnancy, the body needs additional omega-3 fatty acids to promote the growth and development of the baby.

There are three forms of omega-3 fatty acids: **Eicosapentaenoic acid (EPA), Docosahexaenoic acid (DHA), and Alpha-linolenic acid (ALA) (ALA).** EPA and DHA are found in fatty fish such as salmon, tuna, and sardines, whereas ALA is found in plant-based sources such as flaxseed, chia seeds, and walnuts.

Although it is vital for pregnant women to ingest omega-3 fatty acids, they should also be wary of consuming high amounts of mercury that may be found in some species of fish. The FDA recommended that pregnant women eat 8-12 ounces of low-mercury fish weekly to promote safe pregnancy.

If a pregnant woman does not receive enough omega-3 fatty acids in their diet, they may consider taking a fish oil supplement. The recommended daily intake of omega-3 fatty acids during pregnancy is 200-300 mg of DHA daily. Pregnant women should consult with their healthcare professional about their particular requirements and whether a supplement is essential to promote safe pregnancy.

3.0 Food Planning and Preparation

3.1 How to plan and prepare healthful meals during pregnancy

Preparing and preparing nutritious meals throughout pregnancy is vital to promote a healthy pregnancy and baby. Here are some recommendations on how to plan and cook healthful meals during pregnancy:

Consume a range of foods: Eating various foods from each category is vital to ensure you receive all the required nutrients for a healthy pregnancy.

Select whole foods: Whole foods are little processed and are often more nutrient-dense than processed meals. Select whole grains, fruits, veggies, lean proteins, and healthy fats.

Include protein in every meal: Protein is vital for the growth and development of your kid. Every meal includes lean proteins such as chicken, turkey, fish, tofu, and beans.

Eat healthy fats: Good fats such as avocado, almonds, seeds, and olive oil are vital for embryonic brain development. Add healthy fats to your diet in moderation.

Minimize processed foods and added sugars: Processed foods and added sugars are generally high in calories and poor in nutrients. Minimize your intake of these foods during pregnancy.

Drink lots of water: Keeping hydrated is vital throughout pregnancy. Try to drink at least eight glasses of water every day.

Schedule your meals and snacks: Preparing your meals and snacks ahead of time will assist in guaranteeing that you are enjoying a balanced diet. Employ a meal planner or app to organize your weekly meals and snacks.

Cook at home: Cooking at home enables you to manage the ingredients and nutrition in your meals. Try to cook at home as frequently as possible.

Make healthy substitutes: Use healthy substitutions for unhealthy items in your favourite dishes. For example, use whole wheat flour instead of white flour or Greek yoghurt instead of sour cream.

Take a prenatal vitamin: Even with a healthy diet, receiving all the required nutrients for a successful pregnancy may be challenging. Taking a prenatal vitamin may assist in ensuring that you are receiving all of the nutrients needed for a healthy pregnancy.

By following these recommendations, you may plan and prepare nutritious meals throughout pregnancy to guarantee a healthy pregnancy and a healthy baby.

3.1.1 Consume a range of meals

Consuming various meals throughout pregnancy is vital to ensure that you and your developing baby receive all of the required nutrients for a healthy pregnancy. Multiple foods supply different nutrients.

Therefore, eating a range of foods from all food categories in your diet is crucial.
For example, fruits and vegetables contain critical vitamins and minerals such as C, A, and potassium, while whole grains supply fibre, B vitamins, and minerals like iron and zinc. Lean proteins like chicken, turkey, fish, tofu, and beans supply amino acids, which are the building blocks of protein, and are needed for fetal growth and development.

Adding various foods to your diet also helps minimize boredom with your meals and makes healthy eating more fun. Explore multiple recipes and cuisines to find fresh and healthful meals you and your kid will appreciate.
Remember that some foods should be avoided during pregnancy, such as raw or undercooked meat, seafood with high levels of mercury, and unpasteurized dairy products. Speak to your healthcare professional about any particular dietary concerns or limits you may have.

By consuming various foods from all food groups, you can guarantee that you and your developing baby receive all the required nutrients for a successful pregnancy.

3.1.2 Select complete foods

Eating whole foods throughout pregnancy may give you and your baby critical nutrients. It can help you receive the required vitamins, minerals, and fibre to promote a healthy pregnancy. Whole foods are minimally processed and contain fruits, vegetables, whole grains, lean meats, and healthy fats.

Whole foods are generally nutrient-dense, indicating that they contain high quantities of vitamins and minerals in contrast to their calorie content. For example, a serving of kale includes vitamin C, vitamin K, and vitamin A, as well as iron and calcium. In contrast, a serving of potato chips is primarily empty of calories and bad fats.

While shopping for groceries, concentrate on healthy foods rather than heavily processed meals. Select fresh or frozen fruits and vegetables instead of canned types, and choose whole-grain bread and pasta rather than refined grains. Select lean proteins like chicken, turkey, fish, and tofu and healthy fats like nuts, seeds, and avocados.

Choosing whole meals and supplying critical nutrients may help avoid excessive weight gain during pregnancy, which can raise the risk of problems. Give your kid the most fantastic start possible by concentrating on complete, nutrient-dense meals.

Protein should be included in every meal during pregnancy since it is vital for fetal development and growth. Protein is necessary for tissue growth and repair, including the developing of a baby's organs, muscles, and bones.

Women should eat 75-100 grams of protein daily during pregnancy, based on their unique requirements and weight. It's critical to spread this throughout the day and add protein to every meal and snack.

Lean meats, poultry, fish, eggs, beans, lentils, tofu, nuts, and seeds are all high in protein. Adding these items to your diet may help you reach your daily protein requirements.

Aim to incorporate a source of protein with each meal while meal planning. This may include eggs or Greek yoghurt for breakfast and a salad with chicken or tofu for lunch. The supper might consist of fish or lean meat with beans or lentils. Snacks might contain nuts or seeds and a protein shake prepared with milk or plant-based milk substitutes.

Including protein in each meal may help maintain a healthy pregnancy and ensure that your baby receives the nutrients they need for optimum growth and development.

Healthy fats are essential for both the mother and the fetus during pregnancy. Fats are necessary for the baby's brain and nervous system development and for the mother's body to absorb crucial vitamins and minerals.

Pregnant women should take 20-35% of their daily calories from fats, focusing on healthy fats like monounsaturated and polyunsaturated fats. Avocados, nuts, seeds, fatty seafood, and olive oil are high in these fats.

Saturated and trans fats should be avoided or limited since they raise the risk of problems such as gestational diabetes and high blood pressure. Saturated fats are found in foods such as red meat, butter, and cheese, while trans fats are found in processed meals such as cookies, cakes, and fried foods.

With meal planning, try to incorporate sources of healthy fats in each meal. This may be avocado toast or a smoothie packed with nuts and seeds for breakfast. Lunch may include a salmon salad or a wrap with hummus and vegetables. Dinner can consist of baked salmon or grilled chicken with roasted veggies and a sprinkle of olive oil.

Consuming healthy fats throughout pregnancy may help promote a healthy pregnancy and ensure your baby receives the nutrients needed for optimum growth and development.

Avoiding processed foods and added sugars is crucial to meal planning and preparation during pregnancy. Processed meals are often heavy in salt, preservatives, and bad fats, which may raise the risk of gestational diabetes, high blood pressure, and other issues.

Instead of processed foods, pick whole, natural foods like fruits and vegetables, whole grains, lean proteins, and healthy fats. These foods are high in vitamins, minerals, and other critical components for a healthy pregnancy.

Also, additional sugars should be avoided as much as possible. Excessive sugar consumption may result in excessive weight gain, which increases the risk of difficulties during pregnancy and delivery. Instead of sugary snacks and beverages, choose healthy options like fresh fruits, unsweetened yoghurt, or nuts and seeds.

Pregnant women may guarantee a healthy and balanced diet that delivers all the required nutrients for a successful pregnancy by reducing processed foods and added sweets.

3.1.6 Make a meal and snack plan

Meal and snack planning is essential in creating a healthful diet during pregnancy. It ensures you receive all the nutrients you need in the proper quantities and at the correct times throughout the day.

While preparing meals and snacks, pregnant women should consider the necessary daily consumption of calories, protein, carbs, and fats. It is also essential to include a variety of nutritious foods in your diet, such as fruits, vegetables, whole grains, lean meats, and healthy fats.

Create a weekly meal plan containing a range of nutritious and tasty dishes to simplify meal planning. This may also help you save time and money by enabling you to plan ahead of time for grocery shopping and avoiding last-minute dinner options.

It is also essential to schedule nutritious snacks throughout the day. Snacks may help you keep your blood sugar levels consistent and give you additional nutrients you may need throughout pregnancy. Fresh fruit, nuts and seeds, yoghurt, and whole grain crackers with hummus or nut butter are all nutritious snacks.

Planning your meals and snacks ensures your body receives the nutrition to sustain a healthy pregnancy.

3.1.7 Prepare meals at home

Cooking at home gives you greater control over the ingredients and methods of meal preparation, which is helpful for a healthy pregnancy diet. While cooking at home, you can use high-quality products such as fresh fruits and vegetables, whole grains, and lean meats. You may also avoid harmful additions such as extra salt, sugar, and bad fats.

Cooking at home also allows you to experiment with different tastes and dishes, making maintaining a healthy pregnancy diet easier. Experiment with various spices, herbs, and beneficial cooking methods to add diversity to your meals.

It's also worth mentioning that cooking at home may be a low-cost option for eating healthy when pregnant. Dining out or ordering takeout daily may add up fast and may not necessarily give the most nutritious alternatives. Cooking at home helps you save money while also ensuring that you eat nutritional meals that are beneficial to your pregnancy and general health.

3.1.8 Create nutritious replacements

Incorporating healthy substitutes in your meals and snacks is a straightforward approach to boosting the nutritional content of your pregnant diet. Here are a few beneficial adjustments you can make:

Replace refined grains with whole grains: Instead of white or straight bread, pasta, and rice, choose whole-grain varieties. Whole grains contain more fibre and other essential nutrients to help you have a healthy pregnancy.

Choose lean proteins such as chicken or turkey breast, fish, or vegetarian protein sources such as beans or lentils. These options are lower in saturated fat and contain essential nutrients such as iron and zinc.

Increase your intake of fruits and vegetables: Aim to include a variety of colourful fruits and vegetables in your meals and snacks. They are high in vitamins, minerals, and fibre, which can help with a healthy pregnancy.

Substitute sugary snacks with healthy alternatives: Instead of grabbing sweets or baked goods, go for fresh fruit, almonds, or yoghurt as snacks.

By making these easy choices, you may boost the nutritional content of your meals and snacks without compromising taste or enjoyment.

3.1.9 Drink lots of water.

Keeping hydrated is essential during pregnancy because it aids in the maintenance of amniotic fluid levels, the regulation of body temperature, and the prevention of constipation. Pregnant women should consume at least 8-10 cups (64-80 ounces) of water daily. Herbal teas, fresh fruit juices, and coconut water are all healthy beverage options in addition to water. Caffeine and alcohol-containing drinks should be limited or avoided since they may harm fetal development. Water consumption can also help to lower the risk of premature labour and other pregnancy complications.

Monitoring your water intake and drinking plenty of fluids throughout the day is critical.

Prenatal vitamins are an essential element of a healthy pregnancy diet. Prenatal vitamins are carefully created to supply pregnant women with the vital vitamins and minerals they need to maintain their health and the healthy development of their babies.

Most prenatal vitamins contain folic acid, iron, calcium, vitamin D, and other essential nutrients like vitamins C, E, and zinc. These vitamins and minerals aid in fetal growth and development and prevent common pregnancy complications like neural tube defects and iron deficiency anaemia.

Taking a prenatal vitamin is critical when you find out you're pregnant. Your doctor may recommend a specific brand or type of prenatal vitamin, and you must follow their advice.

In addition to taking prenatal vitamins, it is critical to maintain a healthy and well-balanced diet. Prenatal vitamins are not a replacement for a healthy diet. But rather a supplement to guarantee that you obtain all of the necessary nutrients for a healthy pregnancy.

Consuming nutrient-dense snacks throughout pregnancy is critical to keep up with the body's increasing energy needs. On the other hand, busy schedules and appetites may often lead to unhealthy eating habits. Here are some healthy snack ideas for hectic days:

Fresh fruits are an excellent source of vitamins, minerals, and fibre. They are small enough to fit in a bag or container for a fast and refreshing snack. Apples, oranges, bananas, and grapes are among the examples.

Nuts and seeds: These foods are high in protein, healthy fats, and fibre. They are tiny enough to fit in a small bag and are ideal for a fast snack. Some examples include almonds, walnuts, pumpkin seeds, and sunflower seeds.
Greek yoghurt: High in protein and calcium, Greek yoghurt may be mixed with fruits or nuts for a healthful snack. It's also high in probiotics, which may help with intestinal health.

Hummus with vegetables: Hummus is produced from chickpeas, which are high in protein and fibre. Combine it with veggies such as carrots, cucumbers, or bell peppers for a crisp and healthy snack.

Hard-boiled eggs are a fantastic source of protein that can be readily prepared ahead of time. These may be eaten alone or with whole-grain crackers for a more substantial snack.

Whole-grain crackers are high in fibre and may be coupled with hummus, cheese, or nut butter to make a more satisfying snack.

Smoothies may be created using a range of fruits and vegetables and protein sources such as Greek yoghurt or protein powder. They are simple to make ahead of time and keep in a portable container for a healthy on-the-go snack.

Cheese with whole-grain crackers: Cheese is high in protein and calcium and may be used with whole-grain crackers to make a more substantial snack.

Energy bars: They may be a handy and healthy snack alternative, but they must be low in added sugars and rich in protein and fibre.

Trail mix: The trail mix is high in protein, healthy fats, and fibre. Making it possible using nuts, seeds, dried fruits, and whole-grain cereal or crackers is possible. Nonetheless, choosing a mix that is minimal in added sugars and salt is critical.

4.0 Breakfast Recipes

Breakfast is an important meal of the day, particularly during pregnancy. It might give you the energy to start your day and keep your pregnancy healthy. Here are some breakfast dishes that are both healthful and simple to prepare:

Oatmeal: A simple but healthy breakfast is cooked with milk or almond milk, topped with fresh berries, almonds, and a drizzle of honey.

Smoothie: For a quick and straightforward morning smoothie, combine frozen fruit, spinach or kale, almond milk, and a scoop of protein powder. For added protein, add a teaspoon of peanut butter or Greek yoghurt.

Greek yoghurt parfait: For a healthy and tasty morning parfait, layer Greek yoghurt, fresh fruit, and granola. For added sweetness, use honey or maple syrup.

Scramble an egg with spinach or other veggies and serve on a whole wheat English muffins or toast. For added taste and nutrition, add avocado or cheese.

Vegetable omelette: Combine eggs, milk, and chopped veggies such as spinach, mushrooms, and bell peppers in a mixing bowl. Sauté in a nonstick skillet and serve with whole wheat bread.

Having a balanced and nutritious breakfast during pregnancy may assist in boosting fetal growth and development while also providing the mother with the energy she needs.

4.0.1 Rolled Oatmeal

Here's an oatmeal recipe:

Ingredients:

- 1 pound rolled oats
- 2 cups of water
- 1 teaspoon salt
- a quarter cup of milk (optional)
- Choose your toppings (such as fruits, nuts, seeds, honey, or maple syrup)

Instructions:

1. Bring 2 cups of water and a pinch of salt to a boil in a medium-sized pot.

2. Reduce the heat to low and add 1 cup of rolled oats to the boiling water. Stir now and again.

3. Cook the oats for 5-10 minutes, or until soft and the mixture has thickened to your preferred consistency.

4. Remove the pan from the heat once the oats are done.

5. Stir in 1/4 cup milk to make the oats creamier if desired.

6. Serve hot in bowls with your favourite toppings, such as fresh fruits, nuts, seeds, honey, or maple syrup.

This oatmeal dish is a terrific healthy breakfast choice since it is rich in fibre and low in fat; plus, it is easy to personalize with your favourite toppings.

4.0.2 Smoothie

Smoothies are a popular and easy breakfast choice for pregnant women who are on the go. They may be nutrient-dense and readily tailored to individual taste preferences.

Here are a few pregnancy-friendly smoothie recipes:

Berry Blast Smoothie Mix 1 cup of mixed berries (strawberries, raspberries, and blueberries), 1 banana, 1 cup of unsweetened almond milk, and a handful of spinach in a blender.

Smoothie with Mango and Yogurt: Combine 1 cup of frozen mango chunks, 1 cup of Greek yoghurt, 1 cup of unsweetened almond milk, and 1 tablespoon of honey in a blender.

Smoothie with Peanut Butter and Banana: In a blender, combine 1 banana, 1 tablespoon of natural peanut butter, 1 cup of unsweetened almond milk, and a handful of ice.

Green Goddess Smoothie One cup baby spinach, 1 banana, 1 kiwi, 1 tablespoon chia seeds, 1 cup unsweetened almond milk, and a handful of ice in a blender.

Chocolate Avocado Smoothie One avocado, 1 banana, 1 tablespoon unsweetened cocoa powder, 1 cup unsweetened almond milk, and a handful of ice in a blender.

These smoothies are great for a quick breakfast or as a snack during the day. They are high in fibre, protein, healthy fats, and necessary vitamins and minerals for the mother and the growing child.

4.0.3 Parfait of Greek yoghurt

Greek yoghurt parfait is a tasty and nutritious breakfast choice that can be easily adjusted to suit your tastes. You'll need the following items to prepare a simple Greek yoghurt parfait:

- 1 cup plain Greek yoghurt
- 1/4 cup granola
- 1 fresh fruit cup (such as berries or chopped bananas)
- 1 teaspoon of honey (optional)

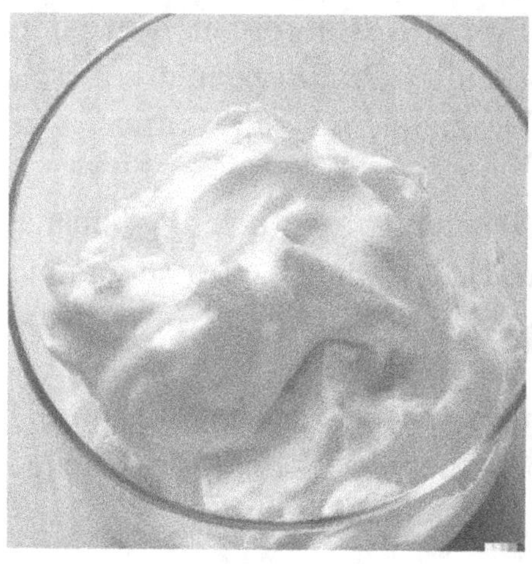

Instructions:

1.   Start by stacking the Greek yoghurt and granola in a bowl or glass. Each layer should include around 1/4 cup of each.

2.   On top of the granola, put fresh fruit.

3. Continue stacking until you reach the top of your bowl or glass.

4. If desired, drizzle honey over the top for extra sweetness.

5. Serve and have fun!

You may also be creative and add more ingredients to your parfait, such as almonds, seeds, or nut butter. This dish is a terrific way to start your day with a healthy and tasty breakfast that will keep you full and energetic all morning.

Here's how to make a tasty and healthy egg sandwich:

Ingredients:

- two huge eggs
- 2 whole wheat bread slices
- 1 tablespoon melted butter
- a quarter cup of shredded cheddar cheese
- Season with salt and pepper to taste.
- Avocado, tomato, or spinach leaves are optional.

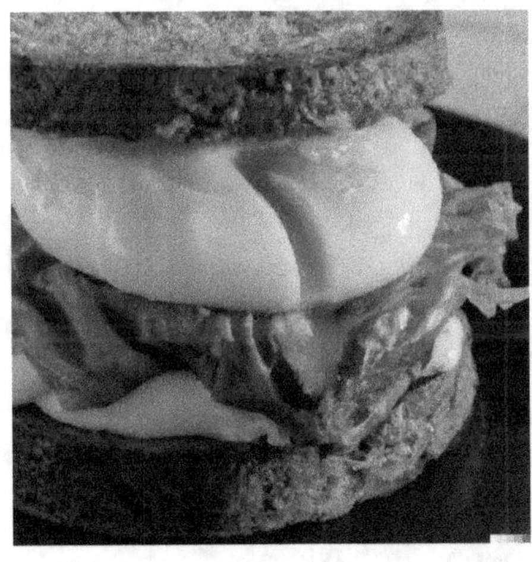

Instructions:

1.	Break the eggs into a mixing dish and whisk until thoroughly combined. Season to taste with salt and pepper.

2.	Melt the butter in a nonstick pan over medium heat.

3.	Scramble the eggs in the skillet until they are cooked through.

4. Toast the bread pieces in a toaster or a pan.

5. Make the sandwich by layering the scrambled eggs on one piece of bread and topping it with shredded cheese. Add extra toppings like avocado, tomato, or spinach leaves if preferred.

Enjoy with the other piece of bread!

This sandwich has an excellent combination of protein, healthy fats, and whole grains, which will keep you satisfied and energetic all morning.

4.0.5 Vegetable Omelette

Here's how to make a vegetarian omelette:

Ingredients:

- 2 eggs
- 1 tablespoon extra virgin olive oil
- 1/4 cup red bell pepper, chopped
- 14 cups finely chopped onion
- 1/4 cup spinach, chopped
- Season with salt and pepper to taste.
- Cheese, shredded (optional)

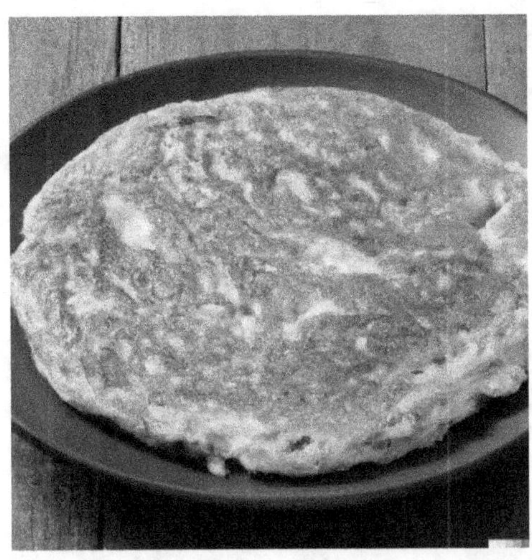

Directions:

1. Whisk the eggs in a small bowl until thoroughly combined.

2. In a nonstick skillet over medium heat, heat the olive oil.

3. Sauté the chopped bell pepper and onion for 2-3 minutes or until softened.

4. Cook for one further minute or until the spinach is wilted.

5. Cook until the eggs start to set, then pour them over the sautéed veggies.

6. Lift the omelette's edges with a spatula to enable the raw eggs to stream below.

7. When the omelette is almost done, top it with shredded cheese (if using).

8. Fold the omelette in half and cook for another minute or until the cheese is melted and the eggs are thoroughly cooked.

Serve immediately and enjoy!

Toast a piece of whole-grain bread and top it with mashed avocado, salt and pepper to taste, and a squeeze of lime juice. Top with sliced tomato, cucumber, or a fried egg for added taste and nutrition.

Chia Seed Pudding: Combine 1/4 cup chia seeds, 1 cup almond milk, and a drizzle of honey in a container. Refrigerate overnight after thoroughly stirring. Before serving, top with fresh berries or sliced bananas.

Scramble 2 eggs with chopped bell peppers, onions, and spinach for a breakfast burrito. Preheat a whole-grain tortilla and top it with scrambled eggs, grated cheese, and salsa or avocado. Roll up your sleeves and enjoy.

Breakfast Quinoa Bowl: Prepare quinoa according to package directions, then add chopped apple, cinnamon, and maple syrup to taste—toasted pecans with a dash of almond milk on top.

These dishes are fast, simple, and full of nutrients to power your morning and start your day correctly.

4.1.1 Toast with Avocado

Avocado toast has recently become a popular and stylish breakfast alternative. It's tasty and high in nutrients, including healthy fats, fibre, and vitamins. Here's a straightforward recipe for avocado toast:

Ingredients:

- 1 avocado, ripe
- 2 whole wheat bread slices
- 1 lime, tiny
- Season with salt and pepper to taste.
- Toppings are optional and include sliced tomatoes, a poached egg, feta cheese, and red pepper flakes.

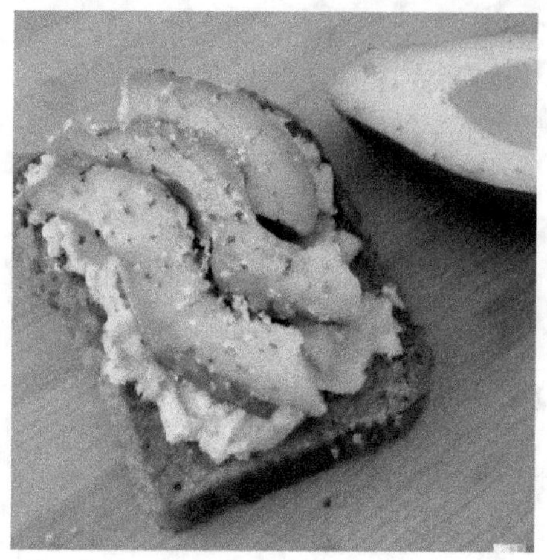

1. Remove the pit from the avocado and cut it in half. Place the meat in a small basin.

2. Using a fork, mash the avocado until it reaches the required consistency.

3. Squeeze the juice of half a lime over the mashed avocado. Combine thoroughly.

4. Toast the bread until it becomes golden brown.

5. Distribute the mashed avocado equally over each piece of bread.

6. Season to taste with salt and pepper.

7. Toppings might include sliced tomatoes, a poached egg, crumbled feta cheese, or a sprinkling of red pepper flakes.

Enjoy your healthy and tasty avocado toast!

4.1.2 Chia Seed Pudding

Chia seed pudding is a healthy and simple breakfast option that can be made the night before, making it an excellent alternative for hectic mornings. Here's how to make chia seed pudding:

Ingredients:

- 1 chia seed cup
- 2 cups almond milk, unsweetened
- 1 to 2 tablespoon honey or maple syrup
- a teaspoon vanilla extract
- Toppings are optional and include fresh fruit, almonds, and shredded coconut.

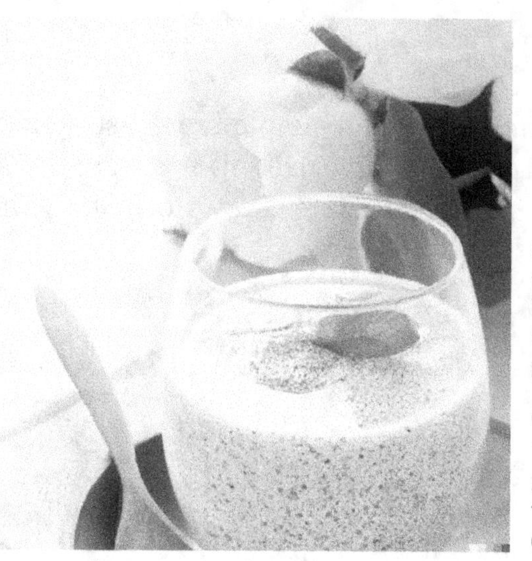

Directions:

1. Combine the chia seeds, almond milk, honey or maple syrup, and vanilla extract in a mixing dish.

2. Refrigerate the dish for at least 4 hours, preferably overnight, to let the chia seeds absorb the liquid and thicken.

3. Give the chia pudding a thorough stir after it has thickened to the desired consistency.

4. Top the chia pudding with your favourite toppings, such as fresh fruit, almonds, or shredded coconut, and serve in bowls or jars.

5. Chia seed pudding is a satisfying and tasty breakfast with fibre, protein, and healthy fats. It may also be modified with various toppings and flavours to suit your tastes.

Here's a recipe for a healthful and straightforward Breakfast Burrito:

Ingredients:

- 1 whole wheat tortilla, big
- 2 eggs
- 1 tablespoon shredded cheddar cheese
- A quarter cup of black beans
- A quarter cup of salsa
- 1/4 sliced avocado
- Season with salt and pepper to taste.

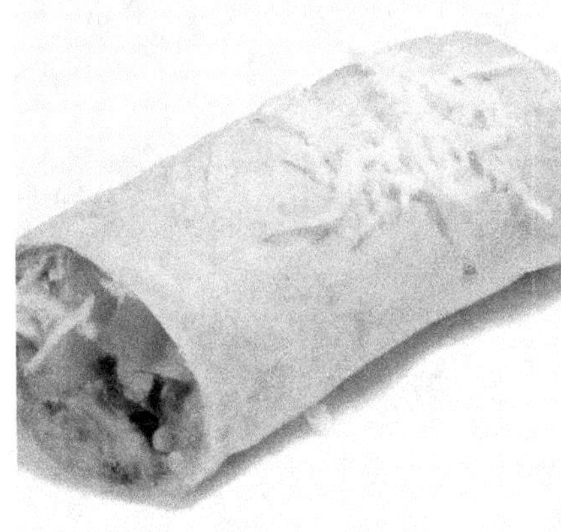

Instructions:

1. Whisk the eggs with salt and pepper in a small bowl.
2. Scramble the eggs in a nonstick pan until they are cooked through.

3. Microwave the tortilla for 10-15 seconds to warm it up.

4. Place the scrambled eggs, black beans, shredded cheddar cheese, salsa, and sliced avocado in the middle of the tortilla.

5. Fold the tortilla's edges over the filling, then it is bottom over it, and roll it up securely.

6. Serve right away.

This morning's burrito has a lot of protein from the eggs and black beans and healthy fats from the avocado. It's a substantial and fulfilling breakfast choice that's easy to personalize with various toppings.

4.1.4 Quinoa Breakfast Bowl

Here's a recipe for a filling and simple morning quinoa bowl:

Ingredients:

- 1 cup quinoa, cooked
- 1/2 cup almond milk, unsweetened
- 1/2 teaspoon cinnamon
- 1 tablespoon of honey or maple syrup
- 1/4 cup nuts, chopped (such as almonds, walnuts, or pecans)

- A quarter cup of dried fruit (such as raisins or cranberries)
- Fruit that is in season (such as sliced banana, berries, or diced apple)

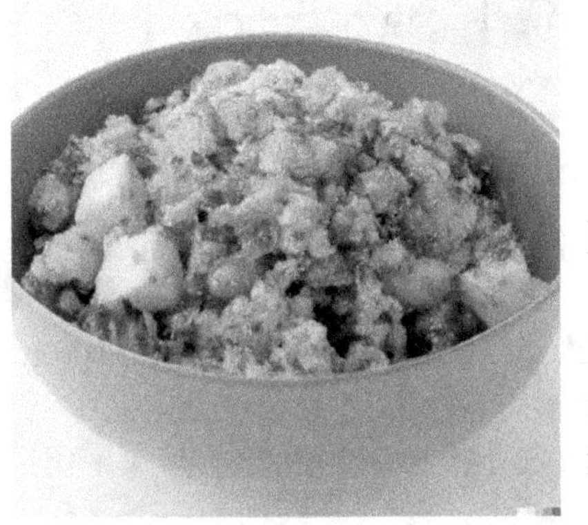

Instructions:

1. Warm the almond milk in a small saucepan over medium heat until warm.

2. Add the cooked quinoa to the pot and mix well.

3. Stir in the cinnamon and honey/maple syrup to mix.

4. Distribute the quinoa mixture evenly between the two dishes.

5. Sprinkle chopped nuts, dried fruit, and fresh fruit on each dish.

Have pleasure in your excellent and healthful morning quinoa dish.

When you're in a hurry in the morning, skipping breakfast entirely is tempting. But beginning your day with a healthy meal is essential, and several meals can be prepared ahead of time or consumed on the move.

Here are some quick and nutritious breakfast alternatives for a hectic morning:

Overnight oats: The night before, combine oats, milk (or a dairy-free substitute), and your favourite toppings (such as fruit, nuts, and honey) in a jar. Grab the pot and go in the morning!

Homemade granola bars: During the weekend, make a batch of granola bars and store them in the fridge for a quick breakfast or snack. Sweeten with honey or maple syrup, oats, almonds, seeds, and dried fruit.

Morning muffins: Prepare a batch of muffins high in healthy grains, fruits, and vegetables. These may be prepared and frozen, then easily reheated in the morning.

Hard-boiled eggs: Make a batch at the start of the week and grab one on your way out the door. For a complete breakfast, serve with fruit or whole-grain bread.
Even on your busiest mornings, there's no need to miss breakfast with these dishes.

For hectic mornings, overnight oats are a quick and nutritious breakfast alternative. Here are a few recipes to get you started:

Traditional Overnight Oatmeal:

Ingredients:

- 1 pound rolled oats
- A half-cup of milk (any kind)
- 1 teaspoon chia seeds
- 1 tablespoon honey (or maple syrup) (optional)
- A half teaspoon of vanilla extract (optional)
- 1 teaspoon salt

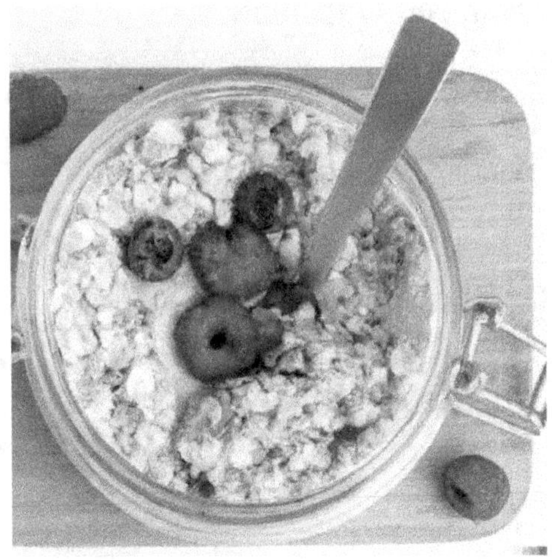

Instructions:

1. Combine all the ingredients in a jar or container with a tight-fitting cover.

2. To blend, stir everything together.

3. Refrigerate overnight, covered.

4. Give the oats a good toss in the morning and top them with your favourite toppings, such as fresh fruit, nuts, or granola.

Overnight Peanut Butter Banana Oatmeal:

Ingredients:

- 1 pound rolled oats
- A half-cup of milk (any kind)
- 1 tablespoon plain Greek yoghurt
- 1 teaspoon chia seeds
- 1 tablespoon. peanut butter
- 1/2 mashed banana
- 1 teaspoon maple syrup or honey (optional)
- 1 teaspoon salt

Instructions:

1. Combine all the ingredients in a jar or container with a tight-fitting cover.

2. To blend, stir everything together.

3. Refrigerate overnight, covered.

4. Give the oats a good toss in the morning and top with more banana slices and a drizzle of peanut butter.

Overnight Blueberry Almond Oatmeal:

Ingredients:

- 1 pound rolled oats
- A half-cup almond milk
- 1 tablespoon plain Greek yoghurt
- 1 teaspoon chia seeds
- 1/2 cup blueberries, fresh
- 1 tablespoon honey (or maple syrup) (optional)
- 1 teaspoon salt

Instructions:

1. Combine all the ingredients in a jar or container with a tight-fitting cover.

2. To blend, stir everything together.

3. Refrigerate overnight, covered.

4. Give the oats a good toss in the morning and sprinkle with more blueberries and sliced almonds.

Overnight Chocolate Banana Oatmeal:

Ingredients:

- 1 pound rolled oats
- A half-cup of milk (any kind)
- 1 tablespoon plain Greek yoghurt
- 1 teaspoon chia seeds
- 1 teaspoon cocoa powder
- 1/2 mashed banana
- 1 teaspoon maple syrup or honey (optional)
- 1 teaspoon salt

Instructions:

1. Combine all the ingredients in a jar or container with a tight-fitting cover.

2. To blend, stir everything together.

3. Refrigerate overnight, covered.

In the morning, give the oats a good toss and top with more banana slices and chocolate powder.

4.2.2 Granola bars created from scratch

Homemade granola bars are a tasty and healthy choice for a quick breakfast or on-the-go snack. They are simple to prepare and may be personalized with several ingredients to suit your tastes. Here are two homemade granola bar recipes:

Recipe 1: Traditional Oatmeal Granola Bars

Ingredients:

- 2 cups oats, old-fashioned
- half a cup of honey
- 1 pound peanut butter (or almond butter)
- 1/4 cup applesauce, unsweetened
- 1/4 cup nuts, chopped (such as almonds or walnuts)
- A quarter cup of dried fruit (such as raisins or cranberries)
- 1/4 teaspoon salt

Instructions:

1. Preheat the oven to 350 degrees Fahrenheit and line an 8x8 inch baking tray with parchment paper.

2. Combine oats, chopped nuts, dried fruit, and salt in a large mixing basin.

3. Microwave honey and peanut butter in a separate dish for 30 seconds or until melted. Mix in the applesauce.

4. Pour the wet components over the dry ingredients and incorporate them well.

5. Fill the prepared baking pan halfway with the mixture and push down firmly.

6. Bake for 20-25 minutes or until the top is golden brown.

7. Let to thoroughly cool before cutting into bars.

Chocolate Chip Granola Bars (Recipe 2)

Ingredients:

- 2 cups oats, old-fashioned
- half a cup of honey
- 1 pound peanut butter (or almond butter)

- 1/4 cup applesauce, unsweetened
- A quarter cup of tiny chocolate chips
- 1/4 cup nuts, chopped (such as almonds or walnuts)
- 1/4 teaspoon salt

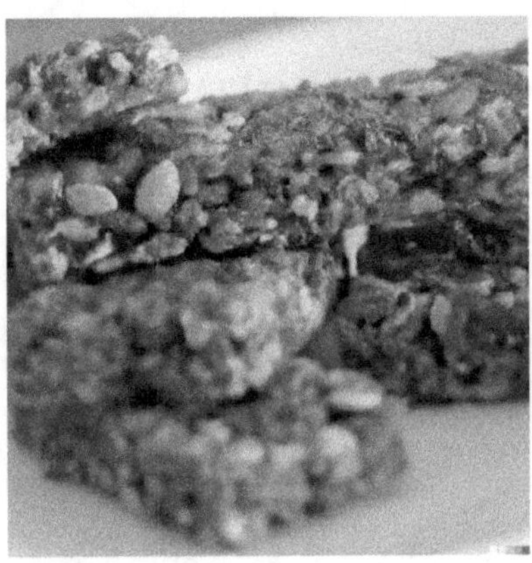

Instructions:

1. Preheat the oven to 350 degrees Fahrenheit and line an 8x8 inch baking tray with parchment paper.

2. Combine oats, chopped almonds, chocolate chips, and salt in a large mixing basin.

3. Microwave honey and peanut butter in a separate dish for 30 seconds or until melted. Mix in the applesauce.

4. Pour the wet components over the dry ingredients and incorporate them well.

5. Fill the prepared baking pan halfway with the mixture and push down firmly.

6. Bake for 20-25 minutes or until the top is golden brown.

7. Let to thoroughly cool before cutting into bars.

4.2.3 Muffins for breakfast

Here are some recipes for healthy and simple breakfast muffins:

Spinach and Feta Egg Muffins:

1. Whisk together 8 eggs, 1 cup chopped spinach, 1/2 cup crumbled feta cheese, 1/4 cup milk, and salt and pepper to taste in a mixing bowl.

2. Fill each muffin cup approximately two-thirds of the way filled with the mixture. Bake for 18-20 minutes until the muffins are firm in the middle, at 350°F.

Blueberry Oatmeal Muffins:

1. Whisk together 1 1/2 cups all-purpose flour, 1 cup rolled oats, 1/2 cup sugar, 2 teaspoons baking powder, 1/2 teaspoon baking soda, and 1/4 teaspoon salt in a large mixing dish. In a separate mixing dish,

combine 1 cup of milk, 1/4 cup of vegetable oil, 1 big egg, and 1 teaspoon of vanilla essence.

2. Mix the wet and dry ingredients until barely mixed. Mix in 1 cup of fresh or frozen blueberries. Bake for 18-20 minutes, or until a toothpick inserted into the middle of a muffin comes out clean, in a greased muffin tray.

Banana Nut Muffins:

1. Whisk together 2 cups of all-purpose flour, 1/2 cup sugar, 2 teaspoons baking powder, 1/2 teaspoon baking soda, and 1/4 teaspoon salt in a large mixing bowl.
2. Mash 2 ripe bananas in a separate basin and combine with 1/2 cup plain Greek yoghurt, 1/4 cup vegetable oil, 2 giant eggs, and 1 teaspoon vanilla essence.
3. Combine the wet and dry ingredients in a mixing bowl.

Till everything is just combined, include 1/2 cup chopped walnuts. Bake for 18-20 minutes, or until a toothpick inserted into the middle of a muffin comes out clean, in a greased muffin tray.

Chocolate Chip Zucchini Muffins,

1. Combine 1 1/2 cups all-purpose flour, 1/2 cup sugar, 2 teaspoons baking powder, 1/2 teaspoon baking

soda, 1/2 teaspoon cinnamon, and 1/4 teaspoon salt in a large mixing bowl. In a separate mixing dish, combine 1 big egg, 1/2 cup milk, 1/4 cup vegetable oil, and 1 teaspoon of vanilla essence. One medium zucchini, grated, should be folded into the wet ingredients. Mix the wet and dry ingredients together until barely mixed. Include 1/2 cup of chocolate chips.

2. Bake for 18-20 minutes, or until a toothpick inserted into the middle of a muffin comes out clean, in a greased muffin tray

4.2.4 Hard-boiled Eggs

Hard-boiled eggs are a healthy and straightforward breakfast choice. These are some hard-boiled egg recipes:

Traditional Hard-Boiled Eggs:

Ingredients:

- Six huge eggs
- Water

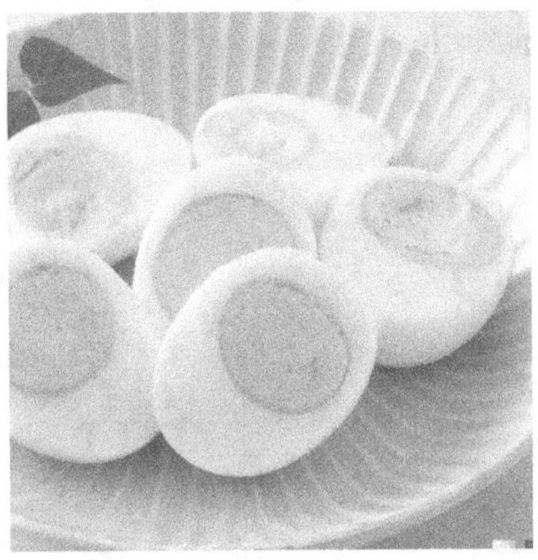

Instructions:

1. Add enough water to cover the eggs in a saucepan.

2. Over medium-high heat, bring the water to a boil.

3. Cover the saucepan from the heat, and set it aside for 12 minutes.

4. Remove the eggs from the boiling water and put them in a dish of ice-cold water for 5 minutes.

5. Serve the eggs peeled.

Toast with avocado and hard-boiled egg:

Ingredients:

- 2 peeled and sliced hard-boiled eggs
- 1 peeled and mashed avocado
- 2 slices whole-wheat bread
- Season with salt and pepper to taste.

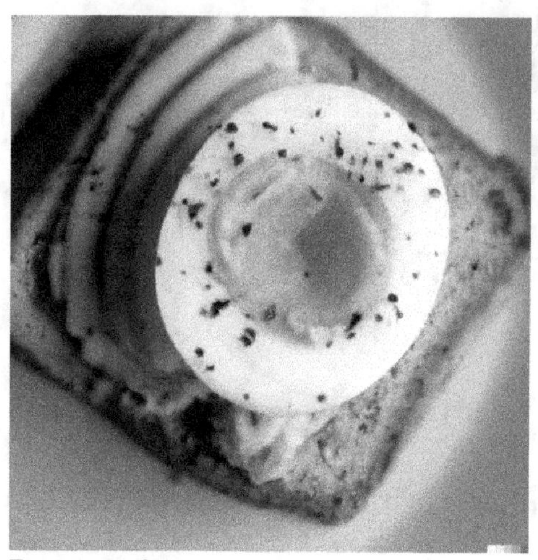

Instructions:

1. Toast the pieces of bread.

2. Distribute the mashed avocado equally across the bread.

3. Top each bread with egg pieces and season with salt and pepper.

Breakfast Cups with Bacon and Eggs:

Ingredients:

- 6 bacon strips
- 6 peeled and sliced hard-boiled eggs
- 1 tablespoon shredded cheddar cheese
- Season with salt and pepper to taste.

Instructions:

1. Preheat the oven to 400 degrees Fahrenheit (200 degrees Celsius).

2. Cooking spray should be used to grease a muffin tray.

3. Each bacon strip should be cut and wrapped around the muffin cup.

4. Fill each muffin cup with a piece of hard-boiled egg.

5. Top each egg piece with grated cheddar cheese.

6. 10-12 minutes, or until the bacon is crispy.

7. Before serving, season with salt and pepper.

These dishes are easy and quick to prepare and can be readily kept in the refrigerator for an on-the-go breakfast.

5.0 Lunch Recipes

5.1 Wholesome and filling lunch alternatives for pregnant women

A healthy and balanced diet is essential for the mother and the growing baby throughout pregnancy. This includes nutritious lunch selections that may supply the nutrients needed for a healthy pregnancy. Here are some ideas for healthy and filling pregnancy lunches:

Salad with Grilled Chicken: Grilled chicken is high in protein and goes well with a range of vegetables, including mixed greens, tomatoes, cucumbers, and carrots. For a healthy fat boost, drizzle with vinaigrette dressing.

Turkey & Avocado Wrap: For a filling and healthy lunch, use a whole grain wrap and fill it with sliced turkey, avocado, lettuce, and tomato. This wrap is high in protein, good fats, and fibre.

Quinoa & Vegetable Bowl: Quinoa is a high-protein grain that pairs well with roasted or sautéed vegetables, including bell peppers, zucchini, onions, and mushrooms. Add a dab of hummus to add protein and a taste boost.

Lentil Soup: Lentils are high in protein and fibre and may be utilized to produce a substantial and filling soup. Season with herbs and spices after adding vegetables such as carrots and celery.

Baked Sweet Potato and Broccoli: Baked sweet potatoes are high in vitamins and minerals, while broccoli is high in fibre and other essential components. For a tasty and healthful meal, roast them together.

Tuna Salad with Whole Grain Crackers: Tuna is high in protein and healthy fats and may be paired with chopped veggies like celery and onion to produce a delightful and filling salad. For a crispy texture, serve with whole-grain crackers.

Vegetable Burger with Sweet Potato Fries: A vegetarian burger cooked with whole grains and veggies is a high-protein, fibre-rich option. Serve with baked sweet potato fries for a wholesome and filling meal.

Here are just a few examples of healthy and filling pregnant lunch alternatives. Ensure that you and your baby receive the required nutrients for a healthy pregnancy, including various fruits, vegetables, whole grains, lean protein, and healthy fats.

Grilled Chicken Salad Recipe with Instructions:

Ingredients:

- 2 skinless, boneless chicken breasts
- Seasoned with salt & pepper
- 1 romaine lettuce head
- 1 diced cucumber
- 1 chopped red bell pepper
- 1/2 sliced red onion
- 1 diced avocado
- 1/4 cup feta cheese, crumbled
- 1/4 cup almonds, sliced
- 2 tablespoon fresh parsley, chopped
- 2 tablespoons olive oil
- 2 tablespoons lemon juice

Instructions:

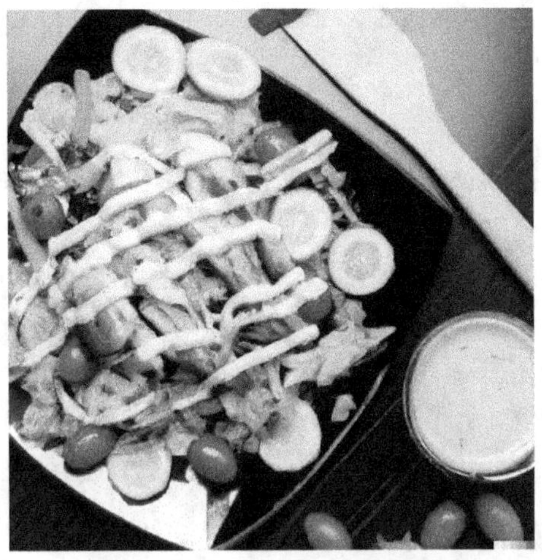

1. Preheat the grill to medium-high temperature—season both sides of the chicken breasts with salt and pepper.

2. Grill the chicken for 6-7 minutes on each side or until done. Let for a 5-minute rest before slicing.

3. Prepare the salad items while the chicken is frying. Wash and dice the lettuce, cucumber and red bell pepper, slice the red onion, and dice the avocado.

4. Mix the olive oil and lemon juice in a small bowl to create the dressing.

5. Salad components should be arranged on a big platter or individual plates.

6. Serve the salad topped with grilled chicken slices.

7. Dress the salad with the dressing.

8. Top with crumbled feta cheese, sliced almonds, and fresh parsley.

Serve and have fun!

Notes:

- For this salad, you may use whatever sort of lettuce you choose.
- Add veggies to the salad, such as cherry tomatoes or shredded carrots.
- You may cook the chicken on the stovetop or in the oven if you don't have a grill.

The dressing may be customized by adding honey, dijon mustard, or other herbs and spices.

5.1.2 Wrap with Turkey and Avocado

Here's a recipe and how-to for a tasty Turkey and Avocado Wrap:

Ingredients:

- 1 big flour tortilla wrap
- 3 roasted turkey breast slices
- 1/2 sliced avocado
- 1/4 cup lettuce, shredded
- 1/4 cup cherry tomatoes, sliced
- 1/4 cup red onion, sliced
- 1 teaspoon of mayonnaise
- 1 tsp. Dijon mustard

- Season with salt and pepper to taste.

Instructions:

1. Begin by gathering your materials. Thinly slice the turkey breast, slice the avocado, and cut the lettuce, cherry tomatoes, and red onion.

2. Mix the mayonnaise and Dijon mustard in a small bowl until thoroughly blended. Season to taste with salt and pepper.

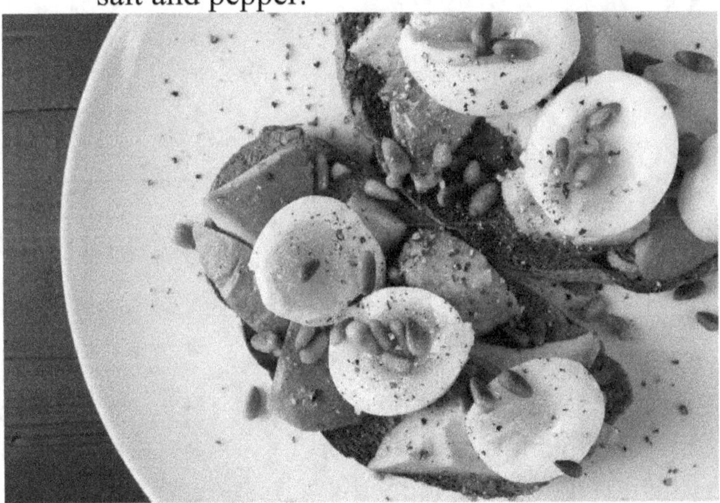

3. Place a clean work surface on top of the tortilla wrap. Distribute the mayonnaise and mustard mixture to the wrap's centre.

4. On top of the mayonnaise and mustard mixture, layer the sliced turkey breast, avocado, shredded lettuce, cherry tomatoes, and red onion.

5. Fold the tortilla's edges towards the centre, then roll up firmly from the bottom, enclosing all the contents.
6. Serve immediately by cutting the wrap in half, or wrap firmly in plastic wrap and chill until ready to eat.

Enjoy your tasty and healthy Turkey and Avocado Wrap!

5.1.3 Bowl with Quinoa and Vegetables

Recipe for Quinoa and Vegetable Bowl

Ingredients:

- 1 cup washed and drained quinoa
- 2 cups veggie broth or water
- 1 chopped red bell pepper
- 1 chopped yellow bell pepper
- 1 small red onion, chopped
- 1 small sliced zucchini
- 1 diced tiny yellow squash
- 1 cup halved cherry tomatoes
- 1 can drain and rinse chickpeas

- 1/4 cup fresh parsley, chopped
- 1/4 cup fresh cilantro, chopped
- 2 tablespoon of olive oil
- 2 tablespoon lemon juice, freshly squeezed
- Season with salt and pepper to taste.

Instructions:

1. Combine quinoa and water or vegetable broth in a medium pot. Bring to a boil, lower to low heat, and cook for 15-20 minutes until all the liquid has been absorbed and the quinoa is fluffy.

2. Preheat the oven to 400°F in the meanwhile. Toss the chopped red and yellow bell peppers, red onion, zucchini, and yellow squash in one tablespoon of olive oil, salt, and pepper. Place the veggies on a baking sheet in a single layer and roast for 15-20 minutes or until soft and slightly browned.
3. Mix the remaining tablespoon of olive oil, lemon juice, salt, and pepper in a small dish to prepare the dressing.

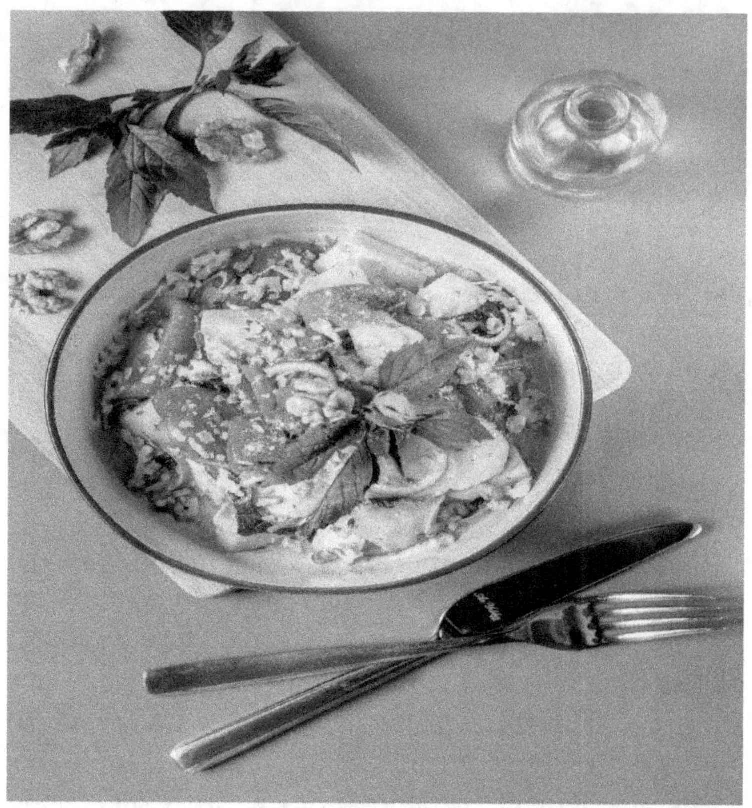

4. Combine the cooked quinoa, roasted veggies, cherry tomatoes, chickpeas, parsley, and cilantro in a large mixing bowl. Drizzle with the dressing and mix everything until thoroughly incorporated.

5. Warm or at room temperature, serve. This dish yields 4 servings.

Note: Add grilled chicken or shrimp to this dish for an added protein boost.

Lentil soup is a nutritious and filling lunch choice that is ideal for pregnant women. Lentils are high in protein, fibre, and other essential elements. Here's a recipe and how-to for a delectable lentil soup:

Ingredients:

- 1 cup washed and drained dry lentils
- 1 chopped onion
- 2 minced garlic cloves
- 2 peeled and sliced carrots
- 2 celery stalks, chopped
- 1 undrained can of chopped tomatoes
- 4 cups broth (vegetable or chicken)
- 1 teaspoon thyme dried
- 1/2 teaspoon rosemary dried
- Season with salt and pepper to taste.
- 1 tablespoon extra virgin olive oil
- Chopped fresh parsley (optional)

Instructions:

1. Warm the olive oil in a big saucepan over medium heat. Mix in the onion, garlic, carrots, and celery. Sauté for 5-7 minutes or until the veggies are tender.

2. Rinse the lentils, then add the chopped tomatoes with juice, vegetable or chicken broth, dry thyme, and rosemary. To blend, stir everything together.

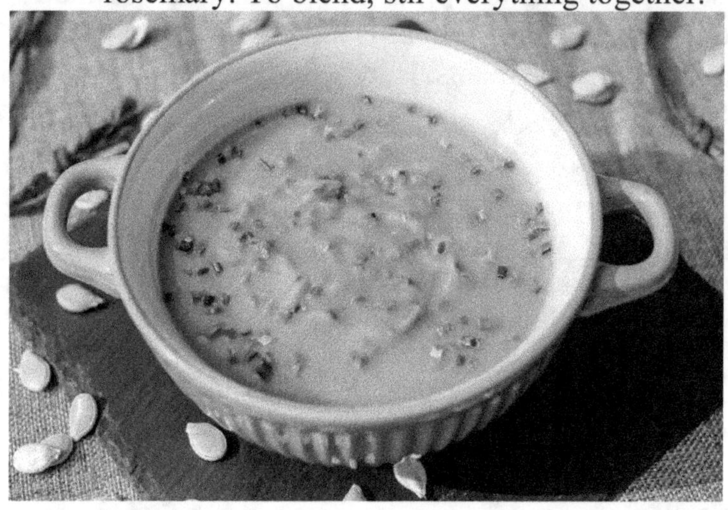

3. Bring the soup to a boil, lower it to low heat and cover. Cook, occasionally stirring, for 20-30 minutes or until the lentils are cooked.

4. Take the soup from the heat and season it to taste with salt and pepper.

5. Serve hot, garnished if desired, with fresh parsley.

This lentil soup is not only healthful and nutritious, but it is also simple to prepare. Make a big batch and keep it in the fridge or freezer for fast and straightforward lunches throughout the week. Enjoy!

Baked Sweet Potato with Broccoli is a tasty and healthful vegetarian meal that can be served for lunch or supper. Here is a detailed recipe and how-to instructions for making this dish:

Ingredients:

- Two medium sweet potatoes
- 2 cups florets broccoli
- 1/2 cup red onion, chopped
- 2 minced garlic cloves
- 1 tablespoon extra virgin olive oil
- 1 teaspoon thyme dried
- Paprika, 1/2 teaspoon
- Season with salt and pepper to taste.

Instructions:

1. Preheat the oven to 400 degrees Fahrenheit (200 degrees Celsius) and line a baking sheet with parchment paper.

2. Wash the sweet potatoes and poke them with a fork many times. Bake for 45-50 minutes, or until they are soft, on a baking sheet.

3. Meanwhile, combine the broccoli florets, chopped onion, minced garlic, olive oil, dried thyme, paprika, salt, and pepper in a mixing dish.

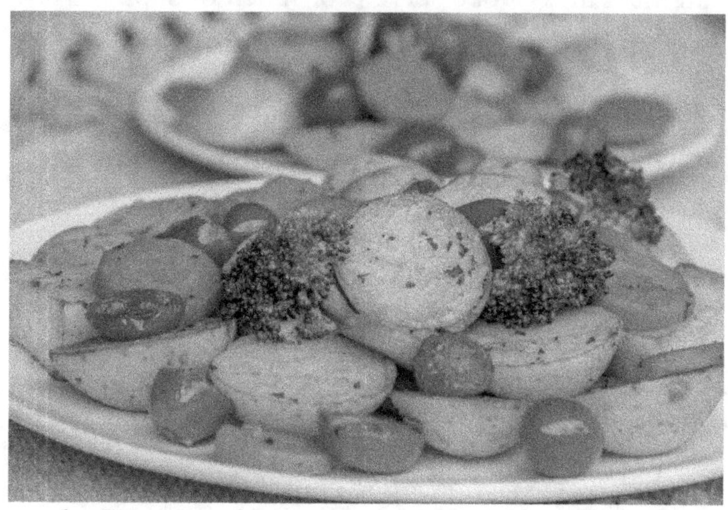

4. Remove the sweet potatoes from the oven and set aside for a few minutes to cool.

5. Scoop off part of the meat from the sweet potatoes to form a cavity for the broccoli mixture.

6. Fill each half of a sweet potato with the broccoli mixture.

7. Bake the sweet potatoes for 15-20 minutes or until the broccoli is soft and gently browned.

8. Remove from the oven and serve immediately.

This recipe is adaptable and may be tailored to your preferences. Other vegetables, such as bell peppers or carrots, may be added to the broccoli combination to add taste and nutrients. You can add protein to the sweet potato halves by topping them with crumbled feta cheese or chopped almonds.

Baked Sweet Potato with Broccoli is a filling and healthy recipe that is simple to prepare and ideal for a fast lunch or supper.

5.1.6 Tuna Salad with Whole Wheat Crackers

Ingredients:

- 1 drained tuna can
- 2 tablespoon unsweetened Greek yoghurt
- 1 teaspoon Dijon mustard
- 1 teaspoon lemon juice
- 1 sliced celery stalk
- 1 little sliced red onion
- Season with salt and pepper to taste.
- Serve with whole-grain crackers.

Instructions:

1. Add the drained tuna to a medium-sized mixing bowl and break it into tiny pieces with a fork.

2. Mix in the plain Greek yoghurt, Dijon mustard, and
   lemon juice until thoroughly blended.

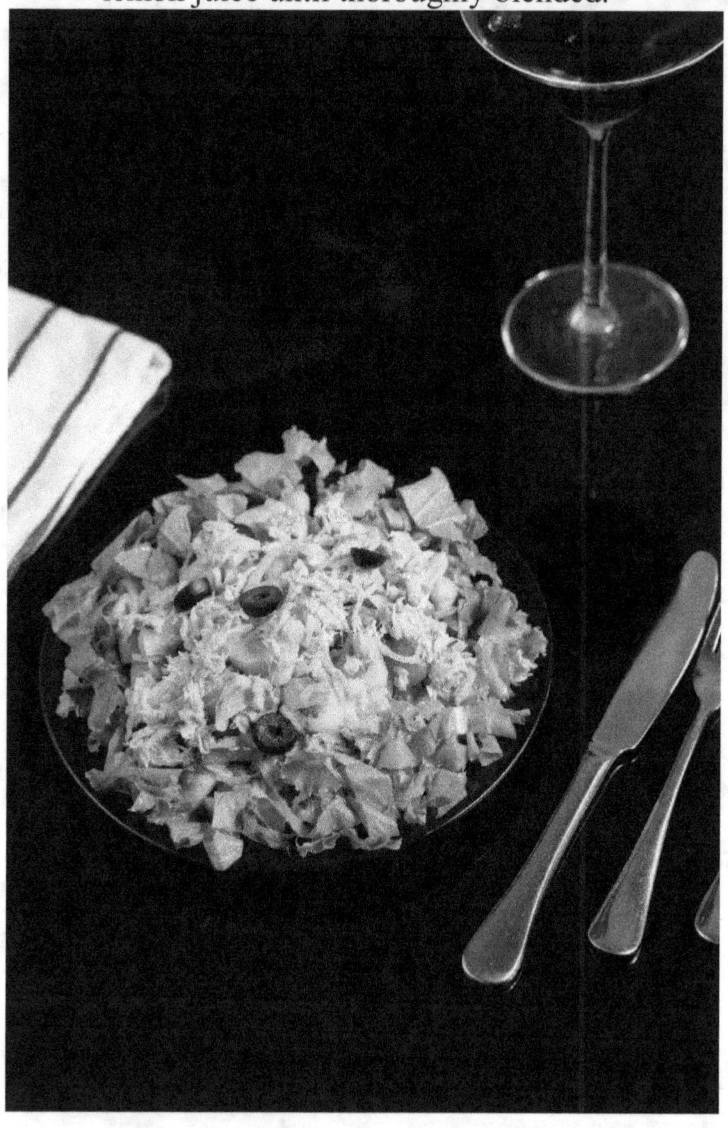

3. Combine the celery and red onion.

4. Season the mixture to taste with salt and pepper.

5. On the side, serve the tuna salad with whole grain crackers.

Notes:

- For sweetness and texture, other ingredients, such as chopped apples or dried cranberries, can be added to the tuna salad.

Store the tuna salad in an airtight container in the fridge for up to 3 days to make it ahead.

Whole grain crackers are a healthy and filling carbohydrate source to complement the protein-rich tuna salad. For extra nutrients and fibre, serve the tuna salad on top of a bed of greens.

5.1.7 Sweet Potato Fries and Veggie Burger

Recipe for a Veggie Burger with Sweet Potato Fries

Ingredients:

1 can (15 ounces) of rinsed and drained black beans

1 cup brown rice, cooked

1 cup whole grain breadcrumbs

1 egg

14 cups finely chopped onion

1/4 cup green bell pepper, chopped

1/4 cup red bell pepper, chopped

a half teaspoon of chilli powder

a half teaspoon of cumin
Season with salt and pepper to taste.
4 whole wheat buns
4 cheddar cheese slices
1 big peeled and sliced sweet potato into fries
1 tablespoon extra virgin olive oil
a half teaspoon of garlic powder
1 tablespoon smoked paprika
Season with salt and pepper to taste.
Instructions:
Preheat the oven to 400 degrees Fahrenheit.
Mash the black beans with a fork or potato masher in a large mixing basin until nearly smooth.
Combine brown rice, breadcrumbs, egg, onion, green bell pepper, red bell pepper, chilli powder, cumin, salt, and pepper in a mixing bowl. Combine everything until thoroughly blended.
Shape the ingredients into four 1/2-inch-thick patties.
Melt butter in a nonstick pan over medium heat. Cook for 3-4 minutes on each side or until the patties are browned.
Place the patties on a baking sheet lined with parchment paper. Put a piece of cheddar cheese on top of each cake and bake for 5-10 minutes or until the cheese has melted.
Prepare the sweet potato fries while the burgers are baking. Toss the sweet potato fries with olive oil, garlic powder, smoked paprika, salt, and pepper in a mixing bowl.
Place the sweet potato fries on a baking sheet in a single layer and bake for 20-25 minutes or until crispy and golden brown.

Place each burger patty on a whole grain bun and top with your preferred burger toppings before serving. On the side, fill in the sweet potato fries.

Take pleasure in your handmade vegetarian burger and sweet potato fries!

5.2 Lunchtime Meal Prep Recipes

Meal planning is an excellent method to save time and money while eating healthy and nutritious meals throughout the week. Here are some midday meal prep dishes that are both simple to create and wonderful to eat:

Stir-Fry Chicken and Vegetables: In a wok, combine soy sauce, garlic, and ginger with chicken breasts and veggies of your choosing (such as broccoli, carrots, and bell peppers). Serve with brown rice for a filling meal.

Grill or bake chicken breasts and serve with quinoa or brown rice, fresh veggies, and tzatziki sauce in Greek chicken bowls. These bowls may be made with your preferred veggies and toppings.

Mason Jar Salads: In a mason jar, layer your favourite salad components (such as lettuce, tomatoes, cucumbers, and bell peppers), beginning with the dressing at the bottom and ending with the lettuce on top. These salads may be made ahead of time and brought to work for a nutritious and simple lunch.

Wraps with sliced vegetables and hummus: Spread hummus on a whole-grain tortilla (such as cucumbers, carrots, and bell peppers). Fold the tortilla and cut it into bite-sized pieces for a quick and filling meal.

Bowls of Beef with Broccoli: In a wok, cook flank beef and broccoli with garlic, ginger, soy sauce, and honey. For a protein-packed lunch, serve over brown rice or quinoa.

Stuffed Bell Peppers with Turkey and Quinoa: Remove the tops and seeds from the bell peppers. Cooked ground turkey, quinoa, and diced veggies enter the centre. Bake for a nutritious and tasty lunch.

Roasted Vegetable Pasta Salad: Roast veggies in the oven with olive oil and garlic (such as zucchini, bell peppers, and cherry tomatoes). Mix with cooked whole-grain spaghetti and a homemade vinaigrette for a filling meal.

Tuna Salad Lettuce Wraps: Combine canned tuna, Greek yoghurt, chopped celery, and lemon juice in a mixing bowl. For a light and refreshing meal, serve atop lettuce leaves.

These meal prep recipes may be tailored to your preferences and dietary constraints, and they can be kept in the fridge for several days for quick grab-and-go lunches.

Chicken and vegetable stir-fry is a tasty and nutritious dish that can be cooked in a short period. This meal serves four and takes around 30 minutes to make.

Ingredients:

- 1 pound boneless, skinless chicken breasts, thinly sliced
- 1 sliced red bell pepper
- 1 sliced yellow bell pepper
- 1 sliced zucchini
- 1 chopped little onion
- 2 minced garlic cloves
- 2 tablespoons soy sauce
- 2 tablespoons hoisin sauce
- 1 teaspoon cornstarch
- 1 teaspoon sesame oil
- 2 tablespoons vegetable oil
- Season with salt and pepper to taste.
- Steamed rice to serve

Instructions:

1. Whisk together the soy sauce, hoisin sauce, cornstarch, and sesame oil in a small bowl. Set aside.

2. Heat the vegetable oil in a large wok or pan over medium-high heat. Stir-fry the chicken until it is cooked, approximately 5-7 minutes.

3. Stir in the garlic, onion, bell peppers, and zucchini for another 2-3 minutes or until the veggies are tender-crisp.

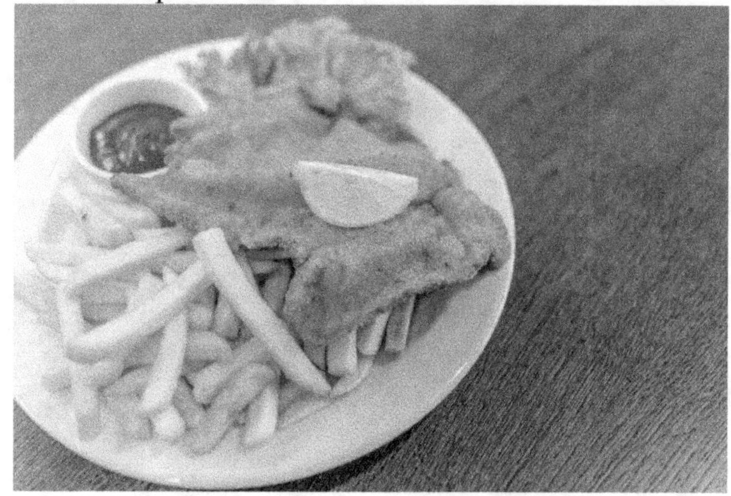

4. Stir the soy sauce mixture into the chicken and veggies to coat. Simmer for another 1-2 minutes or until the sauce has thickened and the veggies have been covered.

5. Season to taste with salt and pepper.

6. Serve the stir-fried chicken and vegetables over steamed rice.

Enjoy your tasty and nutritious chicken and vegetable stir-fry!

5.2.2. Bowls of Greek Chicken

Greek Chicken Bowls are a tasty and nutritious lunch option that is simple to make and ideal for meal preparation. This recipe is high in protein, veggies, and healthy fats, making it filling and healthy.
Here's how to make Greek Chicken Bowls:

Ingredients:

- 1 pound skinless, boneless chicken breasts
- 2 tablespoon of olive oil
- 1 teaspoon of lemon juice
- 1 tablespoon. red wine vinegar
- 1 tablespoon. dried oregano
- 1 teaspoon. garlic powder
- 1 teaspoon sea salt
- 1/2 teaspoon ground black pepper
- 2 cups quinoa, cooked
- 2 cups mixed chopped veggies (such as bell peppers, cucumbers, cherry tomatoes, and red onions)
- 1/2 cup feta cheese, crumbled
- 1/4 cup kalamata olives, pitted
- Serving Tzatziki sauce (optional)

Instructions:

1. Preheat the oven to 375 degrees Fahrenheit.

2. Whisk the olive oil, lemon juice, red wine vinegar, oregano, garlic powder, salt, and pepper in a small bowl.

3. Place the chicken in a baking dish, and cut it into bite-sized pieces. Stir the marinade into the chicken to coat it.

4. Bake for 20-25 minutes or until the chicken is cooked through.

5. Split the quinoa into four meal prep containers.

6. Cooked chicken, chopped veggies, crumbled feta cheese, and kalamata olives go on top of the quinoa.

7. If wanted, serve with tzatziki sauce on the side.

8. Refrigerate the meal prep containers for up to four days.

This recipe is simple to adapt to your tastes. You may use whatever vegetable you choose, and you can adjust the quantities as required. To make it vegetarian or vegan, replace the quinoa with rice or another grain and the chicken with tofu or another protein source. Enjoy!

Mason jar salads are an excellent option for a quick and easy lunch. They're also great for meal prep because you can make a bunch at once and keep them in the fridge for a few days.

Here are a few tasty and healthful Mason jar salad recipes:

Salad with Greek dressing

- 1/4 cup balsamic vinaigrette
- 1/4 cup cucumber, sliced
- 1 tablespoon cherry tomatoes
- 1/4 cup feta cheese, crumbled
- 1/4 cup red onion, sliced
- 1/4 cup kalamata olives, sliced
- 2 cups romaine lettuce, chopped

Layer the ingredients in the above order in a quart-sized Mason jar, beginning with the dressing on the bottom. Place the chopped romaine on top of the pot.
Place the lettuce in a jar, lock it, and place it in the refrigerator until ready to eat.

Salad with tacos

- A quarter cup of salsa
- A quarter cup of black beans

- 1/4 cup bell peppers, chopped
- 1/4 cup avocado, chopped
- 1 tablespoon shredded cheddar cheese
- 2 cups lettuce, chopped

Arrange the ingredients in the above order in a quart-sized Mason jar, beginning with the salsa on the bottom. Cover with the chopped lettuce, seal the pot, and refrigerate until ready to consume.

Salad with chicken Caesar

- 1/4 cup Caesar salad dressing
- 1 tablespoon cherry tomatoes
- 1/4 cup cucumber, sliced
- 1 tablespoon croutons
- 1/4 cup parmesan cheese, shaved
- 2 cups romaine lettuce, chopped
- 4 ounces chopped cooked chicken breast

Layer the ingredients in the above order in a quart-sized Mason jar, beginning with the dressing on the bottom. Cover with the chopped romaine lettuce and diced chicken, seal the pot, and chill until ready to eat.

- 1 tablespoon ranch dressing
- 1/4 cup bacon, diced
- 1/4 cup blue cheese crumbles
- 1 tablespoon cherry tomatoes
- 1/4 cup avocado, chopped
- 2 cups romaine lettuce, chopped
- 4 ounces chopped cooked chicken breast
- 1 sliced hard-boiled egg

Layer the ingredients in the above order in a quart-sized Mason jar, beginning with the dressing on the bottom. Cover with the chopped romaine lettuce, diced chicken, and chopped egg, then seal and chill until ready to serve.

These Mason jar salads are tasty but also healthful and straightforward to prepare. They're ideal for anybody looking for a fast lunch or who wants to eat healthily on the run.

Here's how to make Vegetable and Hummus Wraps:

Ingredients:

- 4 whole grain tortillas
- 1 hummus cup
- 1 sliced red bell pepper
- 1 sliced yellow bell pepper
- 1 sliced zucchini
- 1/2 sliced red onion
- 1/2 cup crumbled feta cheese
- 1/4 cup fresh parsley, chopped
- Season with salt and pepper to taste.

Instructions:

1. Melt butter in a large pan over medium heat. Drizzle with olive oil before adding the cut bell peppers, zucchini, and red onion. Sauté until the veggies are soft and slightly browned, approximately 5-7 minutes. Season to taste with salt and pepper.

2. Warm the tortillas in the microwave or over medium heat in a pan.

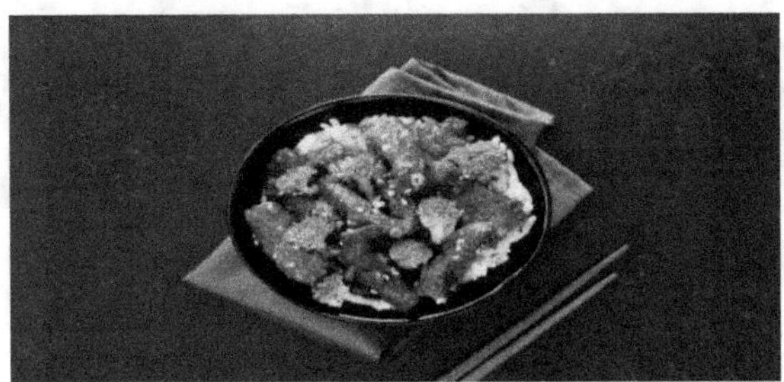

3. Put a good quantity of hummus on each tortilla.

4. Add a couple of spoonfuls of cooked veggies to each tortilla.

5. Crumbled feta cheese and fresh parsley should be sprinkled on each wrap.

6. Before serving, roll the tortillas firmly and cut them in half.

These vegetable and hummus wraps are ideal for a nutritious and filling lunch. You may also make them your own by adding your favourite veggies and herbs. They're also perfect for meal planning ahead of time since they can be kept in the fridge and consumed throughout the week.

Here's how to make Beef and Broccoli Bowls:

Ingredients:

- 1 lb. thinly cut against the grain flank steak
- 3 cups florets broccoli
- 1 sliced red bell pepper
- 1/2 cup onion, sliced
- 2 minced garlic cloves
- 2 tbsp. extra virgin olive oil
- Season with salt and pepper to taste.
- Serve with cooked rice or quinoa.
- Topping: sesame seeds

To make the marinade:

- 1 tablespoon soy sauce
- 2 tbsp. cornstarch
- 2 tbsp. water
- 1 tbsp. honey
- 1 tbsp. sesame seed oil
- 1/2 tsp. ginger, grated
- 1/2 tsp. Flakes of red pepper

Instructions:

1. Whisk together all of the marinade ingredients in a small bowl. Toss in the cut flank steak to coat. Let the steak marinate for at least 30 minutes in the refrigerator.

2. Heat 1 tablespoon olive oil over medium-high heat in a large pan or wok. Cook for 2-3 minutes on each side until the flank steak is browned and cooked. Set the steak aside after removing it from the pan.

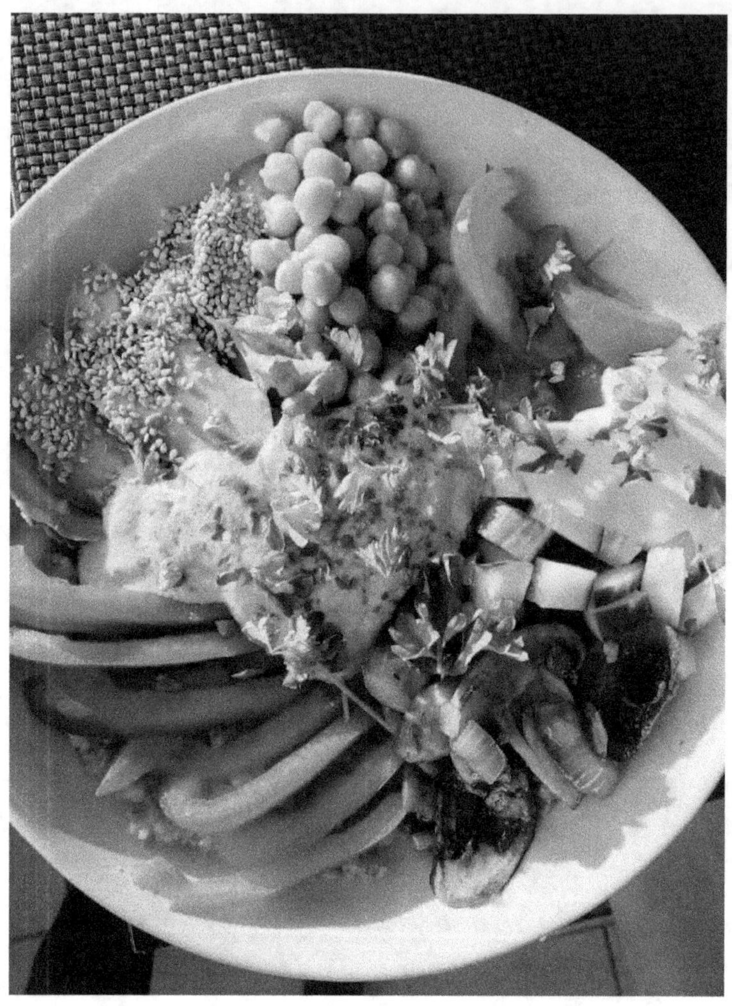

3. Add another tablespoon of olive oil to the same skillet. Combine the sliced bell pepper, onion, and minced garlic in a mixing bowl. Sauté until the veggies are soft, about 2-3 minutes.

4. Cook the broccoli florets in the pan for 2-3 minutes or until they are bright green and tender.

5. Return the cooked steak to the pan with the veggies, stirring to incorporate.

6. Serve the meat and broccoli combination over rice or quinoa that has been cooked. To finish, sprinkle with sesame seeds.

This dish is ideal for meal prep since the beef and broccoli combination can be portioned with rice or quinoa for a hearty and fulfilling lunch.

5.2.6 Stuffed Peppers with Turkey and Quinoa

Turkey and Quinoa Stuffed Peppers are tasty and nutritious dishes that can be served for lunch or supper. Here's a detailed recipe and how-to instructions to help you cook this dish:

Ingredients:

- Four bell peppers
- 1 pound turkey ground
- 1 cup quinoa, cooked
- 1/2 cup finely chopped onion
- 1/2 cup diced tomatoes
- 1/2 cup mushrooms, chopped

- 1 pound shredded cheese
- 1 tablespoon extra virgin olive oil
- Season with salt and pepper to taste.

Instructions:

1. Preheat the oven to 375 degrees Fahrenheit (190 degrees Celsius).

3. Remove the bell pepper tops and remove the seeds and membranes.

4. In a pan over medium-high heat, heat the olive oil.

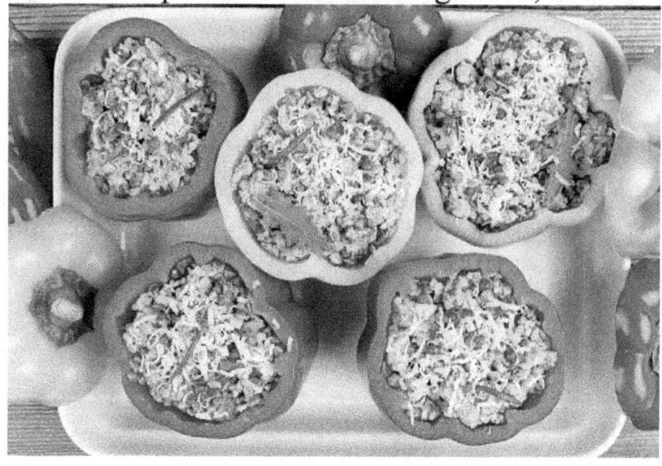

5. Cook for another 2-3 minutes or until the onion is transparent.

6. Cook in the skillet for 5-7 minutes or until the ground turkey is browned.

7. Cook for another 2-3 minutes after adding the chopped tomatoes and mushrooms to the skillet.

8. Stir in the cooked quinoa in the skillet.

9. Season the mixture to taste with salt and pepper.

10. Fill the bell peppers halfway with the turkey-quinoa mixture.

11. Top each filled pepper with shredded cheese.

12. Bake the filled peppers for 25-30 minutes, or until the peppers are soft and the cheese has melted, in a baking dish.

13. Take the filled peppers from the oven and set aside for a few minutes to cool before serving.

14. Enjoy your tasty and filling Turkey and Quinoa Stuffed Peppers!

This recipe for Roasted Vegetable Pasta Salad is ideal for midday meal prep:

Ingredients:

- 1 pound spaghetti (your choice of shape)
- 2 bell peppers, cut into bite-size pieces
- 2 zucchini, cut into bite-sized chunks
- 1 red onion, cut into small bits
- 2 tbsp of olive oil
- Season with salt and pepper to taste.
- 1/2 cup black olives, sliced
- 1/4 cup fresh basil, chopped
- 1/4 cup fresh parsley, chopped
- 1/4 cup feta cheese, crumbled
- To make the dressing:
- 1 tablespoon olive oil
- 1 tablespoon red wine vinegar
- 1 tbsp. Dijon mustard
- 1 minced garlic clove
- Season with salt and pepper to taste.

Instructions:

1. Preheat the oven to 425 degrees Fahrenheit.

2. Toss the diced bell peppers, zucchini, and red onion
    with olive oil, salt, and pepper in a large mixing bowl.

3. Roast the veggies in a single layer on a baking sheet
    for 20-25 minutes, tossing periodically, until soft and
    gently browned.

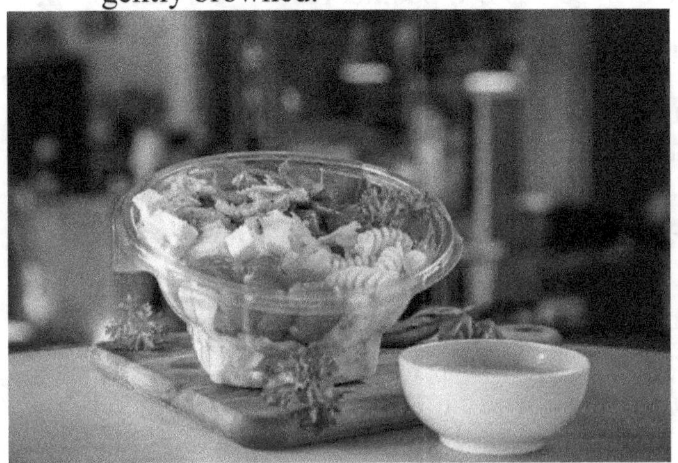

4. Cook the pasta according to package instructions
    while the veggies roast. Rinse with cold water after
    draining.

5. Mix the olive oil, red wine vinegar, Dijon mustard,
    garlic, salt, and pepper in a small mixing bowl to
    prepare the dressing.

6. Combine the cooked pasta, roasted veggies, black
    olives, basil, and parsley in a large mixing basin.

7. Toss the salad with the dressing to mix.

8. Sprinkle with the crumbled feta cheese and serve.

9. This dish serves 6-8 people, making it ideal for meal prep. It's a nutritious, tasty lunch choice packed with veggies and easily modified to your taste preferences. You may also make it vegetarian by omitting the feta cheese or substituting a vegan equivalent.

5.2.8 Lettuce Wraps with Tuna Salad

Tuna salad lettuce wraps are a nutritious and tasty lunch alternative that is quick to make and ideal for meal preparation. Traditional ingredients include canned tuna, Greek yoghurt, mayonnaise, celery, onion, lemon juice, and seasoning. For a low-carb and gluten-free variant, the tuna salad is wrapped in big lettuce leaves such as romaine or butter.

Here's how to make tuna salad lettuce wraps step by step:

Ingredients:

- 2 tuna cans in water, drained
- a quarter cup of Greek yoghurt
- 1 tablespoon mayonnaise
- 1/4 cup celery, finely chopped

- 1/4 cup finely diced onion
- 1 tablespoon freshly squeezed lemon juice
- Season with salt and pepper to taste.
- Romaine or butter lettuce has large lettuce leaves.

Instructions:

- Combine the drained tuna, Greek yoghurt, mayonnaise, celery, onion, lemon juice, salt, and pepper in a medium-sized mixing bowl.

- Arrange the lettuce leaves on a flat surface after washing and drying them.

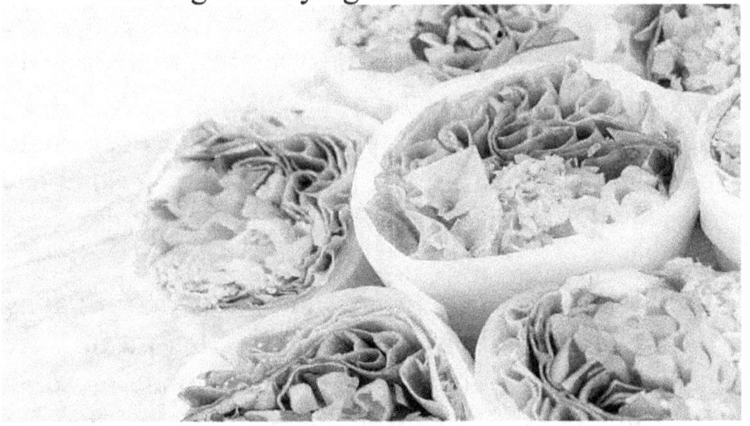

- Place a few teaspoons of tuna salad in the middle of each lettuce leaf.

- Tuck in the sides as you wrap the lettuce leaves around the tuna salad.

- To carry the wraps, secure them using toothpicks or cover them in plastic wrap.

- These tuna salad lettuce wraps may be prepared ahead of time and refrigerated for a fast and straightforward lunch choice all week. These may also be modified with extra vegetables or toppings like avocado, cucumber, or tomato.

- Ivy was overjoyed when she discovered she was expecting. As a health-conscious person, she understood that her diet must adapt to support her developing kid. I wanted to ensure I got all the nutrients for a healthy pregnancy. She decided to begin food preparing her lunches to ensure that she was always eating healthy and fulfilling meals.

- Ivy looked into healthy and tasty ideas for midday meal planning. She wanted to ensure her meals were healthy and straightforward to prepare and preserve for a few days. She experimented with a few recipes to discover which ones she liked best.

- Ivy's first dish was quinoa and veggie bowls. She cooked the quinoa before adding veggies such as bell peppers, tomatoes, and cucumbers. She topped the bowls with feta cheese and a simple olive oil and lemon juice dressing. This meal hit Ivy since it was hearty and high in protein and fibre.

- Ivy then chose to make turkey and quinoa stuffed peppers. She cooked the quinoa and turkey together before seasoning them with herbs and spices. She removed the peppers' tops and scooped out the seeds. She then packed the peppers with the quinoa and turkey mixture and cooked them until soft. This meal was a hit with Ivy since it was a unique way to eat turkey and quinoa, and the peppers gave a wonderful crunch.

- Ivy also tried her hand at preparing salads in mason jars. She started with a layer of veggies, such as kale, spinach, and cherry tomatoes, and then added a layer of protein, such as grilled chicken or hard-boiled eggs. She then covered it with a layer of grains, such as quinoa or brown rice, and a simple vinaigrette. She liked this meal since it was simple to prepare and portable, allowing her to take it to work or errands.

- Ivy experimented with numerous recipes for midday meal prep during her pregnancy. She discovered that planning her meals saved her time and helped her maintain a balanced diet. Ivy's pregnancy was a success, giving birth to a healthy baby boy. She continued to make the dishes she found throughout her pregnancy, and they became regulars in her dinner rotation.

- Ivy reflected on her pregnancy experience and discovered that food preparation was essential to maintaining healthy energy levels. She'd found new and wonderful dishes that she'd enjoyed for years.

6.0 Dinner Recipes

6.1 Pregnancy-Friendly Dinner Recipes

Baked Fish with Roasted Vegetables:

1. Season a salmon fillet with salt, pepper, and olive oil and bake in the oven for 15-20 minutes.

2. Roast your favourite veggies with olive oil and garlic, such as asparagus, carrots, and potatoes.

3. Serve the salmon with the veggies for a satisfying and healthy supper.

Lentil Soup with Whole Wheat Bread: Combine lentils, vegetable broth, chopped tomatoes, onions, garlic, and carrots in a saucepan. Cumin, coriander, and salt to taste. Serve with whole wheat bread for a filling and fibre-rich meal.

Turkey Chili with Brown Rice: In a saucepan, combine ground turkey, diced tomatoes, beans, corn, onions, and garlic: chilli powder, cumin, and salt to taste. Serve with brown rice for a high-protein, satisfying entrée.

Beef Stir-Fry with Brown Rice: Thinly slice meat and stir-fry with broccoli, mushrooms, and bell peppers. Soy sauce, garlic, and ginger to taste. Serve with brown rice for a tasty and nutritious supper.

Chickpea and Sweet Potato Curry: In a saucepan, combine chickpeas and diced sweet potatoes with coconut milk, curry powder, and ginger. Serve with brown rice or quinoa for a delectable vegan supper.
Load large pasta shells with ricotta cheese, spinach, garlic, and parmesan cheese. For a filling and protein-rich supper, top with marinara sauce and bake in the oven.

Grilled Shrimp Skewers with Quinoa Salad: Thread shrimp onto skewers and grill with lemon and garlic until cooked. Serve with a quinoa salad.
Cucumbers, cherry tomatoes, feta cheese, and a lemon vinaigrette dress the salad.

Baked Sweet Potato with Black Beans and Avocado: Bake sweet potatoes with black beans, sliced avocado, salsa, and a dollop of Greek yoghurt. This nutrient-dense vegan dish is ideal for a hectic weekday.

6.1.1 Salmon Baked with Roasted Vegetables

Baked salmon with roasted veggies is a tasty and healthy pregnant meal choice. It is high in protein, healthy fats, and nutrients that benefit the mother and the developing baby. Here's an easy recipe you may make at home:

Ingredients:

- 4 fillets of salmon
- 1 small broccoli head, sliced into florets
- 2 medium peeled and sliced carrots
- 1 sliced red bell pepper
- 1 sliced yellow bell pepper
- 1 tablespoon extra-virgin olive oil
- 1 teaspoon thyme dried
- 1 tsp. garlic powder
- Season with salt and pepper to taste.

Instructions:

1. Preheat the oven to 400 degrees Fahrenheit.

2. Using parchment paper, line a baking sheet.

3. Season the salmon fillets with salt, pepper, and thyme and place them on a baking sheet.

4. Toss the broccoli, carrots, and bell peppers with olive oil and garlic powder in a separate bowl—season with salt and pepper to taste.

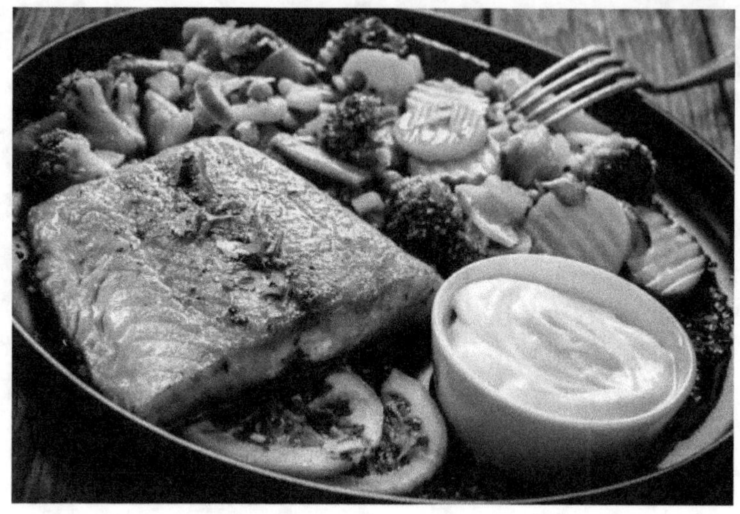

5. Place the veggies on the baking sheet around the salmon fillets.

6. Bake for 15-20 minutes or until the salmon is fully cooked and the veggies are soft.

7. Serve right away and enjoy!

This recipe is not only healthful and tasty, but it is also simple to prepare and ideal for dinner preparation. You may prepare the salmon and veggies ahead of time and then bake them when you're ready to eat. It is an excellent approach to guarantee you receive all the nutrients you need while enjoying a pleasant dinner.

Here's how to make lentil soup with whole wheat bread:

Lentil soup ingredients:

- 1 tablespoon extra virgin olive oil
- 1 chopped onion
- 2 minced garlic cloves
- 2 peeled and sliced carrots
- 2 celery stalks, chopped
- 1 teaspoon cumin powder
- 1 smoked paprika teaspoon
- a quarter teaspoon of cayenne pepper
- 1 cup washed and drained dry green or brown lentils
- 4 cups broth (vegetable or chicken)
- 1 (14.5-ounce) can of undrained diced tomatoes
- 1/4 cup fresh cilantro, chopped
- Season with salt and black pepper to taste.

Whole wheat bread ingredients:

- 1 1/2 cups hot water
- 1 tablespoon dried active yeast
- 1 teaspoon honey
- 1 tablespoon extra virgin olive oil
- 1 teaspoon sea salt
- 3 1/2 cups whole grain flour
- 1 pound rolled oats

Instructions:

1. Heat the olive oil over medium heat in a big saucepan to prepare the lentil soup. Cook for 5 minutes, or until the veggies are soft, with the onion, garlic, carrots, and celery.

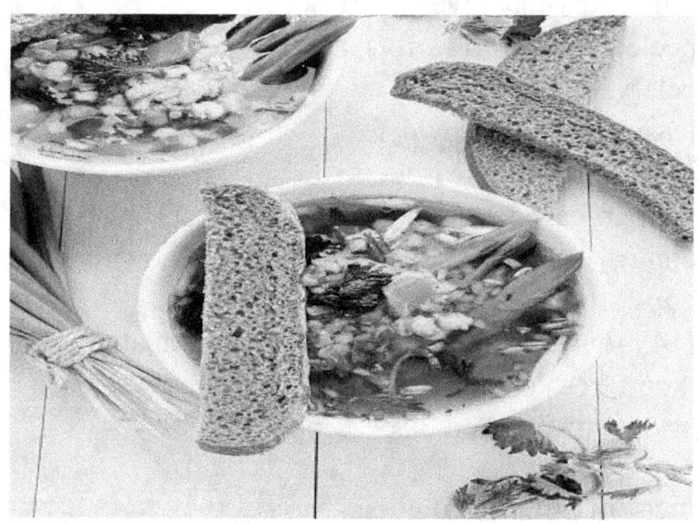

2. Stir in the cumin, smoked paprika, and cayenne pepper until thoroughly combined—Sauté for 1 minute or until aromatic.
3. Pour in the lentils, broth, and chopped tomatoes. Bring to a boil, lower to low heat and continue to cook for 30–35 minutes or until the lentils are cooked.

4. Season with salt and black pepper to taste after adding the cilantro.

5. Combine the warm water, yeast, honey, olive oil, and salt in a large mixing basin to create whole wheat bread. Stir in the whole wheat flour and rolled oats until a dough forms.

6. Knead the dough for 10 minutes on a floured surface, then put it in an oiled bowl and cover it with a moist cloth. Let it rise for 1 hour in a warm environment.

7. Preheat the oven to 375 degrees Fahrenheit. Squeeze the dough down and form it into a loaf. Let the bread rise for 20 minutes in a greased loaf pan.

8. Bake the bread for 30 to 35 minutes until the crust is golden brown and the bottom sounds hollow when tapped.

9. Serve the lentil soup with whole wheat bread pieces on the side. Enjoy!

This recipe yields 4–6 servings of lentil soup and 1 loaf of whole wheat bread. Leftover soup may be refrigerated for up to 4 days, and leftover bread can be kept at room temperature in an airtight container for up to 3 days.

Here's how to make Turkey Chili with Brown Rice:

Ingredients:

- 1 pound ground turkey
- 1 chopped onion
- 1 chopped green bell pepper
- 1 chopped red bell pepper
- 2 minced garlic cloves
- 1 (14.5 oz) can of chopped tomatoes
- 1 can (15 oz) washed and drained kidney beans
- 1 can (15 oz) washed and drained black beans
- 1 (15 oz) can of tomato sauce
- 1 tablespoon chilli powder
- 1 teaspoon cumin
- 1/2 teaspoon paprika
- Season with salt and pepper to taste.
- 2 cups brown rice, cooked
- Toppings are optional and include shredded cheese, sliced avocado, sour cream, and chopped green onions.

Instructions:

1. Melt the butter in a large saucepan or Dutch oven over medium-high heat. Cook until the ground turkey is browned, breaking it into tiny pieces as it cooks.

2. Add the onion, green and red bell peppers, and garlic to the saucepan. Sauté, occasionally stirring, for 5-7 minutes or until the veggies are soft.

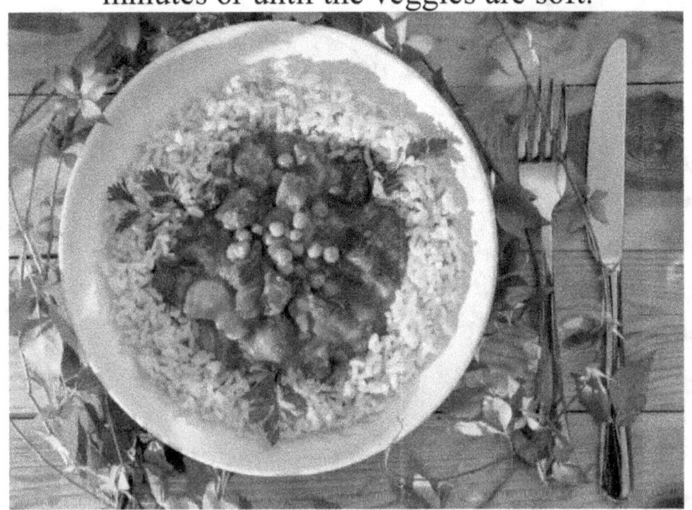

3. In the saucepan, include the chopped tomatoes, kidney beans, black beans, tomato sauce, chilli powder, cumin, paprika, salt, and pepper. To blend, stir everything together.

4. Bring the chilli to a simmer and cook for 20-30 minutes, stirring regularly.
5. Serve the chilli over cooked brown rice with any preferred garnishes.

Enjoy your tasty and filling Turkey Chili with Brown Rice!

Here's how to make Beef Stir-Fry with Brown Rice:
Ingredients:

- 1 lb. cut flank steak into thin pieces
- 2 tbsp. oil from vegetables
- 1 sliced red bell pepper
- 1 sliced green bell pepper
- 1 sliced onion
- 2 minced garlic cloves
- 1 tbsp. minced ginger
- 1 tablespoon soy sauce
- 2 tbsp. honey
- 1 tsp. cornstarch, a quarter cup of beef broth
- Season with salt and pepper to taste.
- 4 cups brown rice, cooked

Instructions:

1. On high heat, heat a big skillet. 1 tsp. Of the vegetable oil.
2. Stir-fry the sliced steak for 2-3 minutes or until browned on both sides. Set the steak aside after removing it from the pan.

3. Mix in the remaining 1 tbsp. Add 1 tablespoon of vegetable oil to the same pan. Stir-fry the sliced bell

peppers and onion for 3-4 minutes or until they soften.

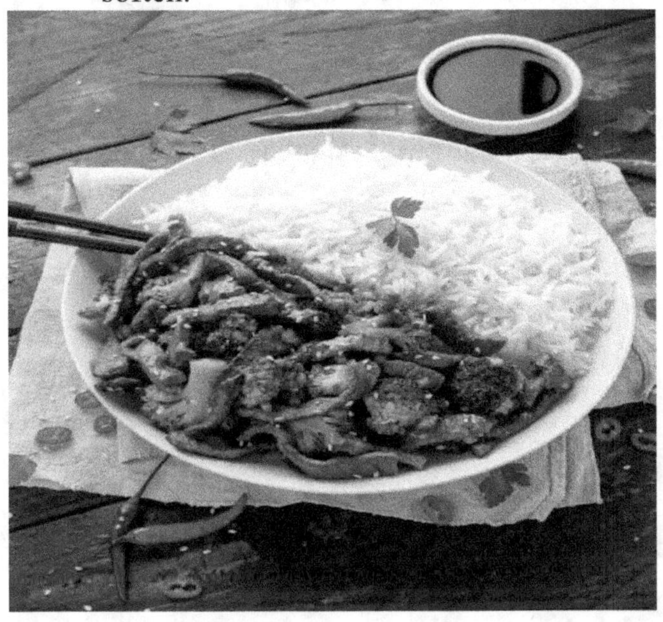

4. Stir in the minced garlic and ginger for a further minute.

5. Combine the soy sauce, honey, cornstarch, and beef broth in a small mixing bowl.

6. Stir the sauce into the veggies in the pan to mix.

7. Return the cooked steak to the pan and stir-fry for another 2-3 minutes, or until the sauce thickens and covers the steak and veggies.

8. Season to taste with salt and pepper.

9. Serve the beef stir-fry with cooked brown rice.

10. Enjoy your tasty and filling Beef Stir-Fry with Brown Rice!

6.1.5 Curry with Chickpeas and Sweet Potatoes

Here's how to make Chickpea and Sweet Potato Curry:

Ingredients:

- 1 tablespoon extra-virgin olive oil
- 1 chopped onion
- 2 minced garlic cloves
- 1 tbsp. grated ginger
- 1 teaspoon curry powder
- 1/2 teaspoon cumin powder
- 1/4 teaspoon cinnamon powder
- 1/4 teaspoon coriander powder
- 2 peeled and sliced sweet potatoes into 1-inch chunks
- 1 can drain and rinse chickpeas
- 1 can chopped tomatoes, drained
- 1/2 cup veggie broth or water
- Season with salt and pepper to taste.
- 2 cups brown rice, cooked

- chopped fresh cilantro (optional)

Instructions:

1. Heat the olive oil over medium heat in a large saucepan or Dutch oven.

2. Cook until the onion is softened, approximately 5 minutes.

3. Cook for another minute after adding the garlic and ginger.

4. Cook for 1-2 minutes or until the curry powder, cumin, cinnamon, and coriander are aromatic.

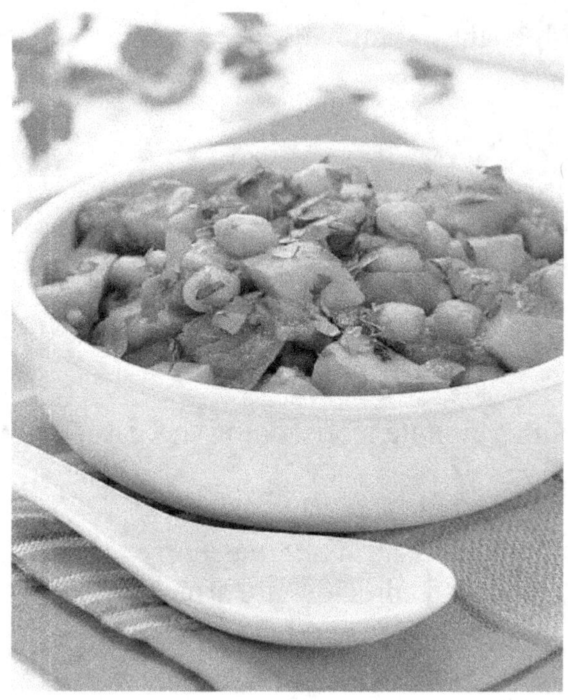

5. Stir in the sweet potatoes and chickpeas to mix with the spices.

6. Stir chopped tomatoes, juice, and water or vegetable broth from the can. To blend, stir everything together.

7. Bring the mixture to a boil, lower to low heat, and cook for 20-25 minutes until the sweet potatoes are soft and the curry thickens.

8. Season the curry to taste with salt and pepper.

9. If preferred, serve the curry over cooked brown rice and garnish with fresh cilantro.

Enjoy your Chickpea and Sweet Potato Curry, which is tasty and healthy!

Here's how to make Spinach and Ricotta Stuffed Shells:

Ingredients:

- 1 giant pasta shells box
- 1 cup ricotta cheese
- 1 1/2 cups thawed and drained frozen spinach
- 1 egg
- 1/2 cup shredded Parmesan cheese
- half a teaspoon of garlic powder
- Season with salt and pepper to taste.
- 2 quarts marinara sauce
- 1/2 cup mozzarella cheese, shredded

Instructions:

1. Preheat the oven to 375 degrees Fahrenheit (190 degrees Celsius).

2. Cook the pasta shells as directed on the box. Set aside
   after draining.

3. Combine the ricotta cheese, spinach, egg, Parmesan
   cheese, garlic powder, salt, and pepper in a mixing
   bowl. Combine thoroughly.

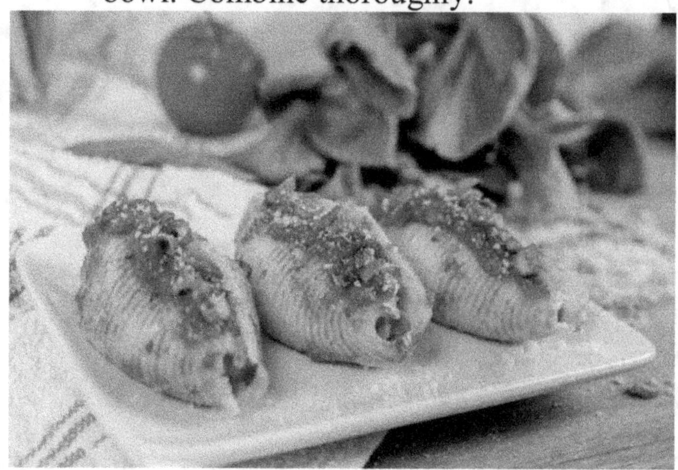

4. Cover the bottom of a 9x13-inch baking dish with
   marinara sauce.

5. Place each shell in the baking dish and fill it with a
   tablespoon of the ricotta and spinach mixture. Rep till
   all of the shots is complete.

6. Spoon the leftover marinara sauce over the shells,
   covering them completely.

7. Top the sauce with the shredded mozzarella cheese.

8. Cover the baking dish with aluminium foil and bake for 30 minutes in a preheated oven.

9. Remove the cover and continue baking for another 10-15 minutes or until the cheese is melted and bubbling.

10. Let the filled shells cool slightly before serving.

Have fun with your Spinach and Ricotta Stuffed Shells!

6.1.7 Grilled Shrimp Skewers with Quinoa Salad:

Here's how to make Grilled Shrimp Skewers with Quinoa Salad:

Ingredients:

- 1 lb. huge peeled and deveined shrimp
- 1 red bell pepper, cut into small bits
- 1 green bell pepper, cut into small bits
- 1 red onion, sliced into small bits
- Season with salt and pepper to taste.
- 2 tbsp. extra virgin olive oil
- 1 quinoa cup
- 2 cups veggie broth or water
- 1/4 cup fresh parsley, chopped
- 1/4 cup fresh cilantro, chopped

- 1/4 cup fresh mint, chopped
- 1 lemon juice
- Season with salt and pepper to taste.

Instructions:

1. Preheat the grill to medium-high temperature.

2. Toss the shrimp, bell peppers, and red onion with salt, pepper, and olive oil in a mixing bowl.

3. Using skewers, thread the shrimp and veggies.

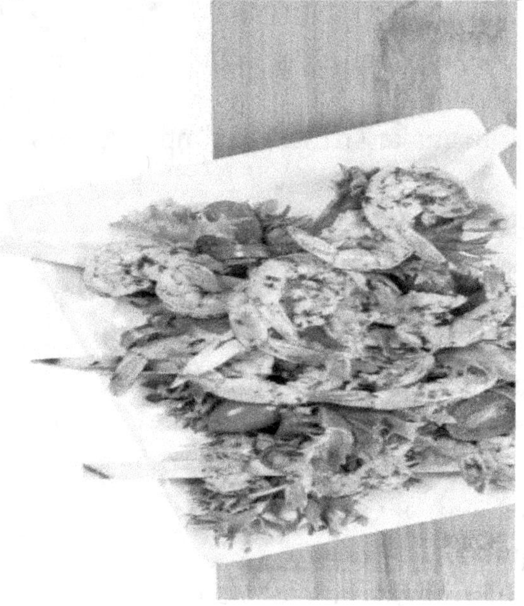

4. Grill the skewers on each side for 2-3 minutes or until the shrimp is pink and cooked.

5. Bring the quinoa and water (or veggie broth) to a boil in a medium saucepan. Lower the heat to low and cook for approximately 15 minutes or until the quinoa is tender and the liquid has been absorbed.

6. Add the cooked quinoa, parsley, cilantro, mint, lemon juice, salt, and pepper in a large mixing bowl. Combine thoroughly.

7. Serve the quinoa salad with the grilled shrimp skewers on top.

Enjoy your tasty and nutritious Grilled Shrimp Skewers with Quinoa Salad!

6.1.8 Sweet Potato Bake with Black Beans and Avocado

Here's how to make Baked Sweet Potatoes with Black Beans and Avocado:

Ingredients:

- 4 large sweet potatoes
- 1 can black beans, washed and drained
- 1 diced avocado
- 1/4 cup fresh cilantro, chopped
- 1/4 teaspoon cumin powder

- 1 tablespoon smoked paprika
- Season with salt and pepper to taste.

Instructions:

1. Preheat the oven to 400 degrees Fahrenheit (200 degrees Celsius).

2. The sweet potatoes should be washed and scrubbed. Using a fork, pierce each one numerous times.

3. Line a baking sheet with parchment paper or aluminium foil and place the sweet potatoes on it. Bake the sweet potatoes for 45-60 minutes or until soft and readily pierced with a fork.

4. Prepare the black bean and avocado topping while the sweet potatoes are baking. Combine the drained and rinsed black beans, diced avocado, chopped cilantro, cumin, smoked paprika, salt, and pepper in a mixing dish.

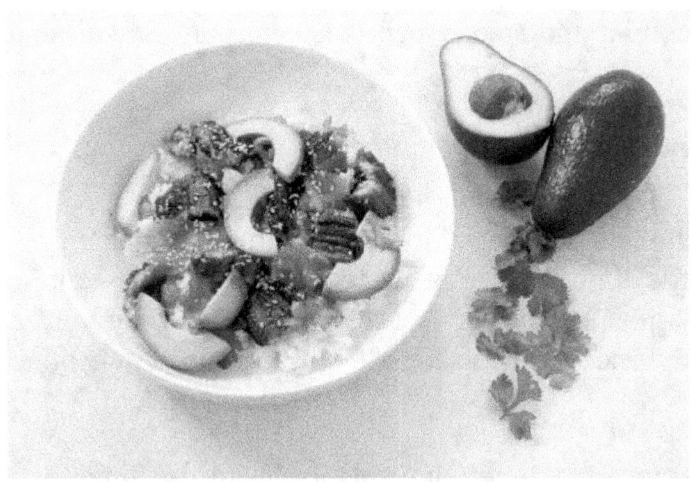

5. Remove the sweet potatoes from the oven and set aside for a few minutes to cool.

6. Cut each sweet potato in half lengthwise and fluff the flesh with a fork.

7. Cover each sweet potato with the black bean and avocado mixture, distributing it equally between them.

8. Serve right away and enjoy!

This recipe is a complete vegetarian alternative that is both tasty and healthful. Sweet potatoes are rich in vitamins and minerals, while black beans are high in protein and fibre. Avocado offers a creamy texture and healthy fats, while cilantro, cumin, and smoky paprika contribute flavour and perfume.

One-pot dinners are ideal for hectic nights when you only have a little time or energy to cook and clean up. These meals take just one pot or pan to prepare, allowing you to spend less time doing dishes and more time doing other things.

Here are some quick one-pot meals for hectic evenings:

One-Pot Pasta: This fast and easy dish only takes one pot and a few ingredients. For a full supper, cook the pasta in a saucepan with veggies and sauce. You may also include protein like chicken, shrimp, or sausage.

One-Pot Chicken and Rice: A traditional one-pot, filling and savoury dish. Brown, add the chicken in a saucepan, then simmer the rice and veggies until the rice is soft and the chicken is well cooked.

One-Pot Chili: A substantial and warm dish ideal for chilly nights. Saute some ground beef or turkey with onions and garlic in a saucepan, then add canned tomatoes, beans, and chilli powder and simmer for approximately 30 minutes.

One-Pot Stir Fry: A fast and healthful supper ideal for hectic nights. Prepare some protein, such as chicken or tofu, with veggies and stir-fry sauce in a saucepan and serve over rice or noodles.

One-Pot Quinoa: This quick and simple dish is high in protein. Prepare some quinoa with veggies and protein, such as chicken or beans, and season with your preferred spices.

One-Pot Roast: This tasty warming dish is ideal for a chilly evening. Cook a roast in a saucepan with onions and garlic, add root vegetables such as carrots and potatoes and bake for a few hours.

One-Pot Casserole: This is a flexible and simple dinner that can be tailored to your preferences. Layer some protein, such as chicken or ground beef, with veggies and grains, such as rice or quinoa, and bake until everything is cooked.

One-pot dinners are ideal for hectic nights since they require little preparation and cleanup and can be tailored to your preferences. They're also excellent for using leftovers while creating fresh and intriguing recipes. Try one of these recipes and see which becomes your new go-to supper for hectic nights.

7.0 Recipes for Snacks

7.1 Healthy Pregnancy Snacks

Healthy snacks are an essential component of a well-balanced pregnancy diet. They may keep you full between meals, give you energy, and guarantee you receive the nutrients you and your developing baby need. Here are some healthy pregnant snack ideas:

Fresh fruit with nut butter: For a protein-packed and fulfilling snack, slice up some apples, pears, or bananas and serve them with a dab of almond or peanut butter.

Greek yoghurt with berries: For a sweet and creamy snack, combine a cup of plain Greek yoghurt with a handful of fresh berries and a drizzle of honey.

Hummus and veggies: For a crunchy and protein-rich snack, cut up some carrots, cucumber, and bell peppers and dip them in a serving of hummus.

Hard-boiled eggs: Cook a batch at the start of the week and store them in the fridge for a quick and protein-rich snack on the fly.

Trail mix: Mix nuts, seeds, and dried fruits for a nutrient-dense snack you can take anywhere.

Roasted chickpeas: Mix chickpeas with olive oil, spices, and a touch of salt and bake for a crispy, protein-packed snack.

Cottage cheese and fruit: For a delicious and protein-rich snack, top a serving of cottage cheese with fresh fruit and a drizzle of honey.

Smoothies: Combine fresh or frozen fruits and vegetables with a scoop of protein powder for a refreshing and nutrient-dense snack.

Whole grain crackers and cheese: Couple an absolute cracker with your favourite cheese for a filling and protein-rich snack.

Remember to pick nutrient-dense foods that will supply you with the energy and nutrition you need to support your developing baby.

7.2 Craving-satisfying recipes

Cravings are usual throughout pregnancy and might be challenging to fulfil healthily. Here are some meals that may satisfy your hunger without losing your nutrition:

Chocolate and Banana Smoothie: Combine 1 ripe banana, 1 tablespoon of chocolate powder, 1 cup of unsweetened almond milk, and 1 teaspoon of honey or agave syrup in a blender.

Greek Yogurt and Berry Parfait: Layer plain Greek yoghurt with berries, granola, and honey drizzle.
Make your own trail mix by combining unsalted nuts (almonds, cashews, and pistachios), dried fruit (cranberries and apricots), and dark chocolate chips.
Thinly slice apples and combine them with cinnamon and honey to make baked apple chips. Bake for 2 hours @ 225°F, turning halfway through.

Sweet Potato Fries: Thinly slice sweet potatoes and mix with olive oil, salt, and paprika. Bake for 20-25 minutes at 425°F, turning halfway through.
To make energy balls, combine 1 cup pitted dates, 1/2 cup rolled oats, 1/2 cup almond butter, 1/4 cup honey, and 1/4 cup dark chocolate chips. Refrigerate after rolling into balls.

Popcorn with Nutritional Yeast: Air-pop popcorn is sprinkled with nutritional yeast for a cheesy taste.
To make Chocolate Avocado Pudding, combine 1 ripe avocado, 1/4 cup chocolate powder, 1/4 cup honey, and 1 teaspoon vanilla extract until smooth.

Guacamole and Vegetable Chips: Combine ripe avocados, lime juice, salt, pepper, chopped tomatoes and onions in a mixing bowl. Dip with vegetable chips or sliced vegetables.

These snacks provide a balanced combination of protein, healthy fats, and complex carbs to satisfy cravings while keeping you full and energetic.

7.2.1 Smoothie with Chocolate and Banana

Here's a tasty and nutritious chocolate and banana smoothie recipe:

Ingredients:

- 1 banana, ripe
- 1 tbsp chocolate powder, unsweetened
- 1/2 cup Greek yoghurt, plain
- 1/2 cup almond milk, unsweetened
- a half teaspoon of vanilla extract
- 1 tbsp honey (or maple syrup) (optional)
- Cubes of ice

Instructions:

1. Place the banana, peeled and sliced, in a blender.
2. In a blender, combine the unsweetened cocoa powder, Greek yoghurt, almond milk, vanilla extract, and honey or maple syrup (if using).

3. Add a handful of ice cubes to the blender to thicken and cool the smoothie.

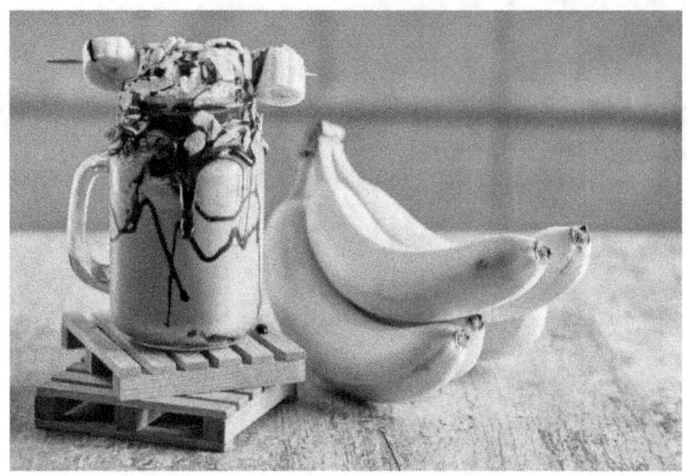

4. Mix all of the ingredients until smooth and creamy.

5. Adjust the sweetness to taste by adding additional honey or maple syrup.

6. Serve the chocolate and banana smoothie immediately in a glass.

Enjoy this tasty and nutritious smoothie as a delightful snack or even a breakfast alternative when pregnant. The chocolate and banana combination gives a natural energy source, while the Greek yoghurt and almond milk provide protein and calcium to meet the requirements of the developing infant.

Homemade trail mix is a healthy and easy snack that you can prepare yourself. To fit your taste preferences, you may build your trail mix with your favourite nuts, seeds, dried fruits, and other items. These are some recipes for homemade trail mix:

Traditional Trail Mix

- 1 cup almonds, toasted
- 1 cup cashews, roasted
- 1 pound of roasted peanuts
- 1 cup dried raisins
- M&M's or chocolate chips, 1 cup

Trail Mix Tropical

- 1 cup chopped dried mango
- 1 cup chopped dried pineapple
- 1 cup coconut flakes, unsweetened
- 1 cup cashews, roasted
- 1 macadamia nut cup

Trail Mix Spicy

- 1 cup almonds, toasted
- 1 cup pistachios, roasted
- 1 cup pumpkin seeds, roasted

* a half-cup of dried cranberries
* 1 tsp. chilli flakes
* 1 tsp. paprika with a smokey flavor
* 1/2 tsp. a pinch of garlic powder
* 1/2 tsp. cumin
* 1/4 tsp. chilli powder
* Trail Mix for Chocolate Addicts
* 1 cup almonds, toasted
* 1 cup cashews, roasted
* 1 cup dipped pretzels in chocolate
* 1 pound chocolate chips
* 1 cup drained dried cherries

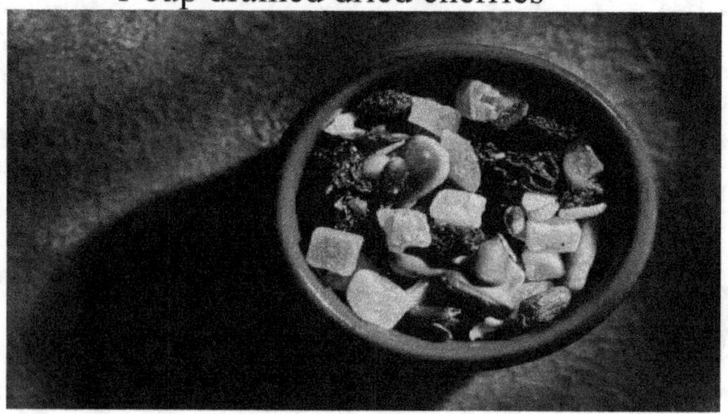

Trail Mix with a Boost of Energy

* 1 cup almonds, toasted
* 1 cup walnuts, toasted
* 1 cup pumpkin seeds, toasted
* 1 cup sunflower seeds, toasted

- Goji berries, 1/2 cup
- 1 pound dark chocolate chips

Combine all ingredients in a dish and store them in an airtight container to prepare any trail mix recipes. Serve as a healthful on-the-go snack or a topping for yoghurt or cereal.

Here's how to make Baked Apple Chips:

Ingredients:

- 2 to 3 big apples
- 1 teaspoon cinnamon powder
- 1 tablespoon granulated sugar
- Spray cooking oil

Directions:

1. Preheat the oven to 225 degrees Fahrenheit (107 degrees Celsius).

2. Wash the apples and use a corer or a sharp knife to remove the core and seeds. Using a mandolin or a sharp knife, thinly slice the apples. Throw away the ends.

3. Combine the ground cinnamon and granulated sugar in a small bowl.

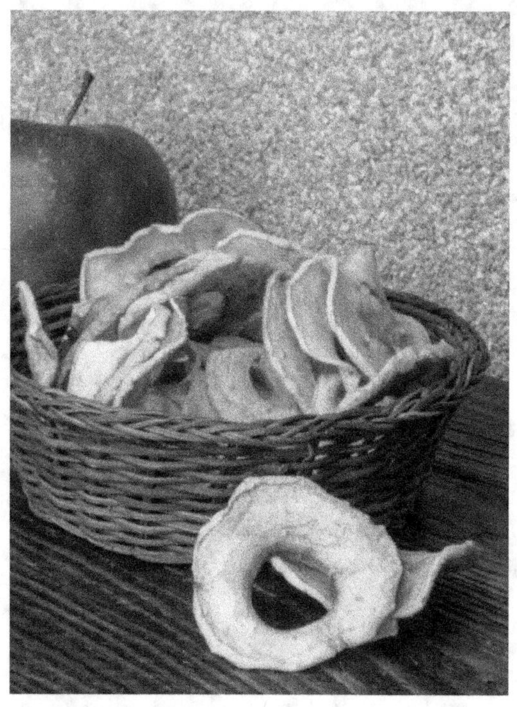

4. Parchment paper or a silicone baking mat line a large baking sheet.

5. Arrange the apple slices in a single layer on the baking sheet. Lightly spray them with cooking spray.

6. Sprinkle the apple slices with the cinnamon-sugar mixture.

7. Bake for 1-2 hours, or until the apple chips are crispy and gently browned, in a preheated oven. Halfway through baking, turn the chips over.

8. When the apple chips are done, take them from the oven and set them aside to cool for a few minutes on the baking sheet. Next, place them on a dish or in an airtight container.

9. These baked apple chips are nutritious and tasty snacks you can prepare at home. These are excellent substitutes for store-bought chips, sometimes rich in salt and preservatives. The richness of the apples complements the cinnamon and sugar wonderfully, making them a delicious treat. Eat them as a snack, or add some crunch to your favourite yoghurt or porridge!

7.2.3 Sweet Potato Fries

Here's how to make sweet potato fries:

Ingredients:

- 2 large sweet potatoes
- 1 tablespoon extra virgin olive oil

- 1 tsp. garlic powder
- 1 paprika teaspoon
- 1 teaspoon of salt
- 1/4 teaspoon ground black pepper

Instructions:

1. Preheat the oven to 425 degrees Fahrenheit (218 degrees Celsius).

2. The sweet potatoes should be washed and peeled.

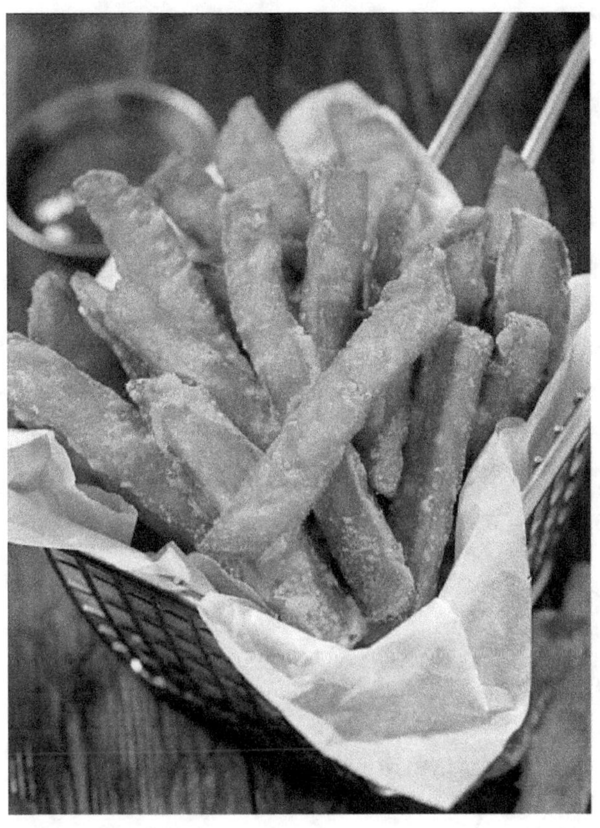

3. Sweet potatoes should be cut into thin, even slices.

4. In a small mixing bowl, combine the olive oil, garlic powder, paprika, salt, and black pepper.

5. Toss the sweet potato strips in the basin with the spice combination until they are well-covered

6. Arrange the sweet potato strips on a baking sheet coated with parchment paper in a single layer.

7. Bake the sweet potato fries for 20-25 minutes, turning halfway through, until crispy and golden brown.

8. Remove from the oven and serve right away.
You may also experiment with other spices and dipping sauces to personalize the taste. Enjoy!

7.2.5 Energy Balls

Here's how to make energy balls:

Ingredients:

- 1 pound rolled oats
- 1 pound almond butter
- 1/3 cup maple syrup or honey
- 1/2 cup coconut flakes
- 1/2 cup nuts, chopped (such as almonds, walnuts, or pecans)
- a quarter cup of dried cranberries
- 1 tablespoon chocolate chips
- 1 tablespoon vanilla extract
- 1 teaspoon salt

Instructions:

1. Combine rolled oats, almond butter, honey or maple syrup, shredded coconut, chopped almonds, dried cranberries, chocolate chips, vanilla essence, and salt in a large mixing dish.

2. Combine all of the ingredients until thoroughly blended.

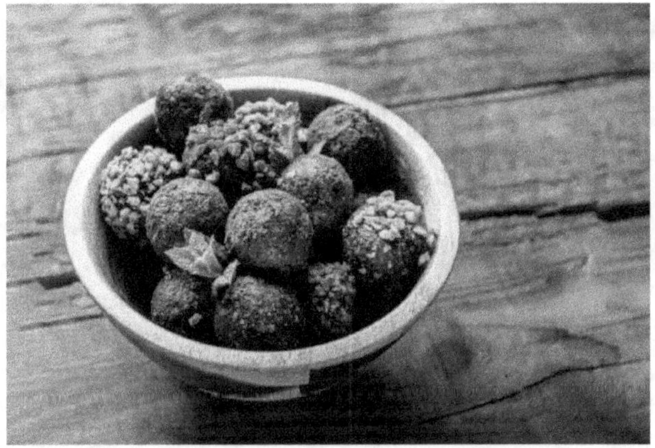

3. Form the dough into 1-inch balls using a cookie scoop or spoon.

4. Refrigerate the energy balls for at least 30 minutes after placing them on a baking sheet lined with parchment paper.

5. After the energy balls have hardened, please place them in an airtight container and refrigerate them for up to one week.

Variations:

1. Substitute almond butter for peanut or cashew butter.

2. To vary the tastes, use a variety of nuts or dried fruit.

3. Add a scoop of protein powder for an additional protein boost.

4. Enjoy these energy balls throughout the day as a fast and pleasant snack!

7.2.6 Chocolate Avocado Pudding

Here's how to make Chocolate Avocado Pudding:

Ingredients:

- 2 pitted and peeled ripe avocados
- 1/2 cup chocolate powder, unsweetened
- 1 tbsp pure maple syrup
- a third of a cup of almond milk (or any other non-dairy milk)
- 1 tablespoon vanilla extract
- 1 teaspoon salt
- Possible garnishes include chopped nuts, sliced fruit, and coconut flakes.

Instructions:

1. Combine the avocados, cocoa powder, maple syrup, almond milk, vanilla extract, and salt in a food processor or blender.

2. Scrape down the sides as required until the mixture is smooth and creamy.

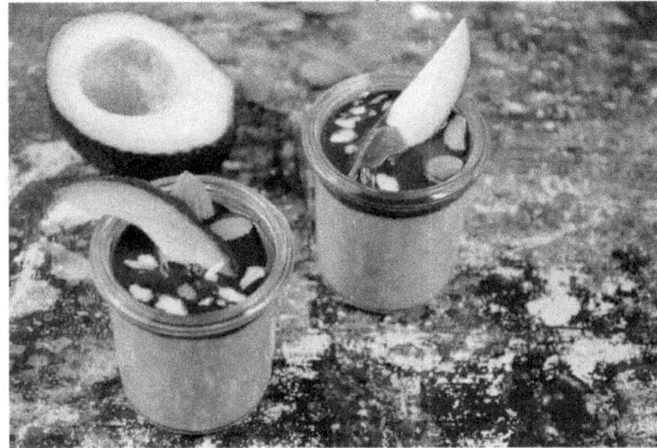

3. Adjust the sweetness with extra maple syrup as desired.

4. Place the pudding in a basin or individual jars to cool.

5. Refrigerate for at least 30 minutes to let it to cold and solidify.
6. Serve chilled with your preferred garnishes.

Enjoy your creamy, decadent, but nutritious Chocolate Avocado Pudding!

Recipe for Nutritional Yeast Popcorn:

Ingredients:

- 1 tablespoon popcorn kernels
- 2 tbsp of coconut oil
- 1 tablespoon nutritional yeast
- a half teaspoon of garlic powder
- a half teaspoon of onion powder
- 1 teaspoon of sea salt
- 1 tablespoon smoked paprika (optional)

Instructions:

1. Over medium-high heat, preheat a big saucepan with a tight-fitting cover. Let the coconut oil melt.

2. Cover the saucepan with the lid and add the popcorn kernels. To avoid burning, shake the pot periodically.
3. After the popping begins, shake the pot periodically until the popping stops. Take the saucepan from the

heat and wait a minute to ensure all kernels have popped.

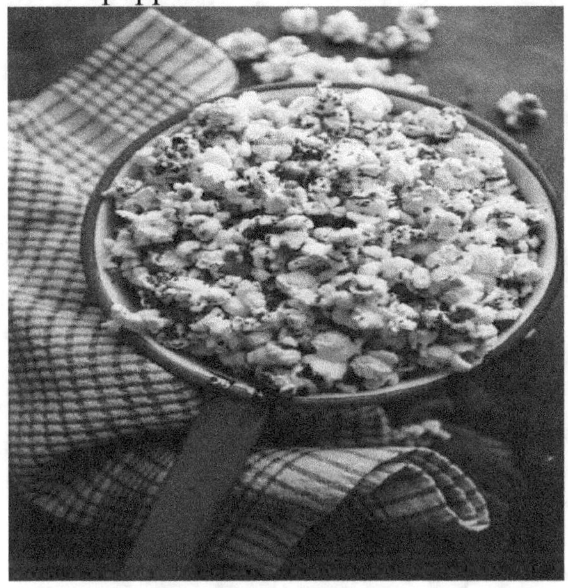

4. Combine the nutritional yeast, garlic powder, onion powder, sea salt, and smoked paprika in a small mixing bowl (if using).

5. Toss the popcorn into a large mixing dish and top it with the nutritional yeast mixture. Stir the popcorn with the seasoning until it is uniformly covered.

6. Serve right away and enjoy!

Nutritional yeast gives the popcorn a cheesy and nutty taste while providing protein and minerals.

Guacamole and Vegetable Chips make an excellent nutritious and filling snack. Here are some suggestions for both:

Guacamole:

Ingredients:

- 2 avocados, ripe

- 1/4 cup onion, chopped
- 1/4 cup tomato, chopped
- 2 tbsp. cilantro, chopped
- 1 minced garlic clove
- One lime juice
- Season with salt and pepper to taste.

Instructions:

1. Remove the pit from the avocados and cut them in half. Place the meat in a mixing basin after scooping it out.

2. Using a fork or potato masher, mash the avocado until it reaches the appropriate consistency.

3. Combine the chopped onion, tomato, cilantro, and garlic in a mixing dish.

4. Squeeze one lime juice over the mixture and season with salt and pepper to taste.

Serve with vegetable chips.

Vegetable Chips:

Ingredients:

- A variety of veggies (such as sweet potatoes, zucchini, carrots, beets, and parsnips)
- Extra virgin olive oil
- seasoned with salt & pepper

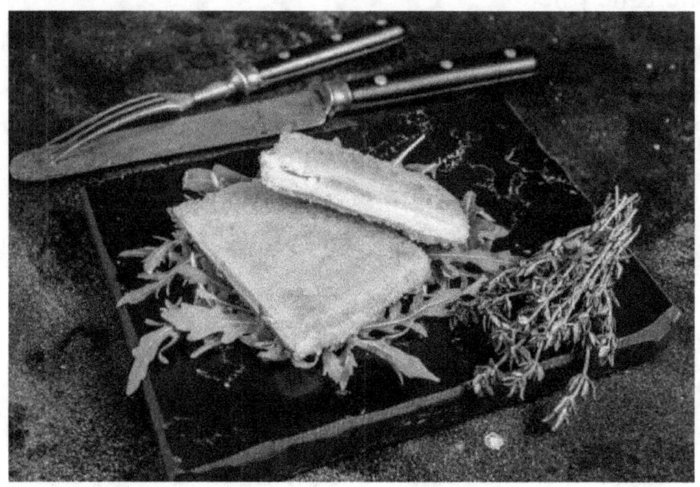

Instructions:

1. Preheat the oven to 375 degrees Fahrenheit.

2. Vegetables should be washed and dried.

3. Slice the veggies into thin rounds using a mandoline or a sharp knife.

4. Drizzle the vegetable slices with olive oil and arrange them on a baking pan in a single layer.

5. Season with salt and pepper to taste.

6. Bake for 15-20 minutes or until golden and crisp.

7. Let to cool before serving with guacamole.

Enjoy your tasty and healthful guacamole and vegetable chips!

8.0 Dessert Recipes

8.1 Pregnancy desserts that are both decadent and healthful

Throughout pregnancy, women must pay special attention to their food to ensure they and their developing baby get all the necessary nutrients. Nonetheless, this does not preclude you from indulging in sweet pleasure. Pregnant women may enjoy a variety of decadent but healthful dessert alternatives. Here are some recipes that fulfil your particular need without jeopardizing your health:

Chia seeds are high in omega-3 fatty acids and fibre, making them a nutritious and complete dessert alternative. In a mixing dish, combine 1/4 cup chia seeds, 1 cup almond milk, 2 teaspoons cocoa powder, and a drizzle of honey to create chocolate chia pudding. Let it rest in the refrigerator for at least 30 minutes before serving.

Baked Apples with Cinnamon: This easy and tasty dish is a great way to satisfy a sweet appetite while obtaining additional vitamins and fibre. Place the slices of an apple on a baking sheet. Sprinkle with cinnamon and bake at 375 degrees Fahrenheit for 10-15 minutes or until the apples are tender and golden.

Banana Oat Cookies: Just three ingredients are used to make these cookies: ripe bananas, rolled oats, and dark chocolate chips. Combine two mashed bananas, 1 1/2 cups rolled oats, and 1/4 cup chocolate chips in a mixing bowl. Scoop the dough onto a baking sheet with a tablespoon and bake at 350 degrees for 12-15 minutes.

Greek Yogurt with Berries and Honey: High in protein and calcium, Greek yoghurt is a nutritious dessert alternative. Top a cup of plain Greek yoghurt with fresh berries and a sprinkle of honey for a tasty and healthy treat.

Frozen Yogurt Bark: This dessert is simple to create and may be personalized with your toppings. Spread 2 cups of plain Greek yoghurt and 1 tablespoon of honey on a baking sheet lined with parchment paper. Freeze for at least 2 hours before breaking into pieces and serving, then top with sliced fruit, nuts, and dark chocolate chips.

Chocolate Avocado Mousse: Since avocado is a good source of fat and fibre, it's an excellent component for a rich and creamy dessert. 2 ripe avocados, 1/4 cup chocolate powder, 1/4 cup maple syrup, and 1/2 cup almond milk, blended until creamy. Refrigerate for at least 30 minutes before serving.

Strawberry Shortcake: Replace classic shortcakes with whole wheat biscuits for a healthy treat. Garnish the biscuits with fresh sliced strawberries, a dollop of Greek yoghurt, and honey whipped cream.

Peanut Butter Banana Ice Cream: Two ingredients are needed for this dessert: frozen bananas and peanut butter. In a blender or food processor, combine two frozen bananas and 2 tablespoons of peanut butter until smooth and creamy. Serve immediately as soft-serve ice cream or place in the freezer for an hour to harden up.

Oatmeal Raisin Cookies: Made with whole wheat flour, oats, and raisins, these cookies are a healthier alternative to classic cookies. In a mixing dish, combine 1 cup whole wheat flour, 1 cup rolled oats, 1/2 cup raisins, 1/2 cup honey, 1/4 cup coconut oil, and 1 egg. Scoop the dough onto a baking sheet with a tablespoon and bake at 350 degrees for 12-15 minutes.

8.2 Special occasion recipes

Here are some ideas for unique occasion recipes:

Prime Rib Roast: This traditional roast is ideal for holidays or special occasions. Serve the roast with roasted veggies and mashed potatoes seasoned with garlic, rosemary, and thyme.

Lobster Risotto: Serve this rich and decadent lobster risotto at a sophisticated dinner party. Creamy arborio rice is cooked with white wine, parmesan cheese, and bits of lobster flesh for dinner, guaranteed to wow.

Chicken Cordon Bleu: Chicken breasts are packed with ham and Swiss cheese, covered with breadcrumbs and cooked till golden brown. Serve with roasted veggies or a side salad.

Beef Wellington: This spectacular recipe is ideal for special occasions. Tender beef fillet is wrapped with prosciutto and mushroom duxelles before being enclosed in puff pastry and cooked till golden and crispy.

Seafood Paella: Serve this traditional seafood paella at a Spanish-themed celebration. This rice dish with shrimp, mussels, clams, and squid is seasoned with saffron and tomato and is ideal for sharing.

Shrimp Scampi: This traditional Italian meal is fast and straightforward yet looks magnificent. Cooked in a garlicky white wine sauce, juicy shrimp are served over linguine.
Grilled Lamb Chops: Grill up some luscious lamb chops for a backyard barbeque or special occasion supper. Before grilling, rub the chops with garlic and rosemary to infuse them with flavour.

Quiche Lorraine: This traditional French meal is ideal for breakfast or a light lunch. A buttery crust is filled with a savoury custard of eggs, cream, and bacon before being baked till golden and fluffy.

Tiramisu: Serve this traditional Italian tiramisu for a sweet and decadent dessert. For a rich and fulfilling dessert, layers of fluffy mascarpone cream and espresso-soaked ladyfingers are topped with chocolate powder.

Here are just a few dishes for special occasions. You may modify these recipes or locate others that fit your requirements depending on your visitors' experience and tastes.

8.2.1 Roast Prime Rib:

Here's how to make Prime Rib Roast:

Ingredients:

- 1 bone-in prime rib roast (4-5 pounds)
- 2 tbsp of olive oil
- 1 tablespoon chopped fresh thyme leaves
- 1 tablespoon chopped fresh rosemary leaves
- 1 teaspoon of kosher salt
- 1 teaspoon black pepper, freshly ground
- 4 minced garlic cloves

Instructions:

1. Remove the prime rib roast from the refrigerator and allow it to come to room temperature for approximately 2 hours before cooking.

2. Preheat the oven to 450 degrees Fahrenheit (232 degrees Celsius).

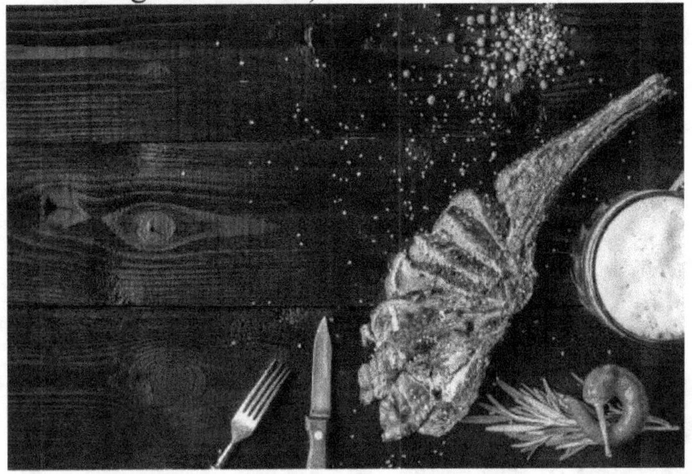

3. In a small bowl, combine the olive oil, thyme, rosemary, salt, pepper, and garlic.

4. The herb combination should be rubbed all over the prime rib roast.

5. Place the roast in a roasting pan with the fat side up.

6. After 15 minutes of roasting, decrease the oven temperature to 350°F (177°C).

7. Cook the prime rib for another 1 1/2 to 2 hours, or until the internal temperature reaches 135°F (57°C)

for medium-rare, 140°F (60°C) for medium, or 150°F (66°C) for medium-well.

8. Take the roast from the oven and set aside 15 minutes before slicing and serving.

Enjoy your succulent prime rib roast!

8.2.2 Risotto with Lobster:

Here's how to make Lobster Risotto:

Ingredients:

- 2 cooked and diced lobster tails
- arborio rice 1 cup
- 1/2 cup white wine, dry
- 3 cups stock (seafood or chicken)
- 1/2 diced onion
- 2 minced garlic cloves
- 2 tbsp of olive oil
- 1/4 cup Parmesan cheese, grated
- 2 tbsp unsweetened butter
- 1 tablespoon fresh parsley, chopped
- Season with salt and pepper to taste.

Instructions:

1. Bring the stock to a simmer in a medium saucepan and keep it warm over low heat.
2. Warm the olive oil in a separate big saucepan over medium heat. Sauté the onion and garlic for 3 minutes or until softened.

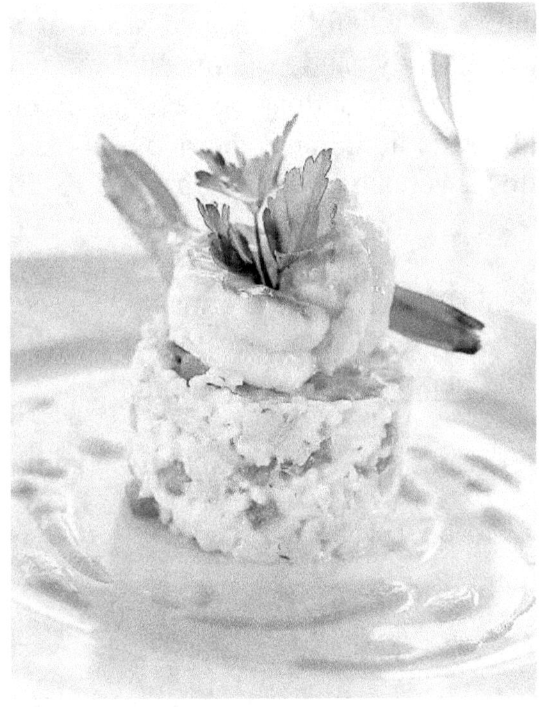

3. Stir the arborio rice in the pot to coat it with the onion and garlic combination. Cook, stirring regularly, for 2 minutes.

4. Pour in the white wine and continue to mix until the rice has absorbed the wine.

5. Begin by adding one ladleful of heated stock at a time, stirring frequently and waiting until each addition is absorbed before adding the next. Continue tossing and adding the liquid until the rice is cooked and the risotto is creamy, approximately 18-20 minutes.

6. Mix in the cooked lobster meat, Parmesan cheese, and butter until well blended and heated. Season to taste with salt and pepper.

7. Serve the lobster risotto immediately, garnished with parsley.

Enjoy your tasty Lobster Risotto!

8.2.3 Cordon Bleu Chicken

Chicken Cordon Bleu is a traditional French cuisine comprising breaded chicken breast packed with ham and cheese, then fried or baked. Here's a recipe you can make at home:

Ingredients:

- 4 skinless, boneless chicken breasts
- four pieces of ham
- 4 Swiss cheese slices
- 1/2 cup regular flour
- 2 beaten eggs
- 1 pound breadcrumbs
- a half teaspoon of garlic powder
- paprika, 1/2 teaspoon
- seasoned with salt & pepper
- 1 tablespoon vegetable oil

Instructions:

1. Preheat the oven to 375 degrees Fahrenheit.

2. Make a pocket in each chicken breast, but don't cut all the way through.

3. Place a piece of ham and a slice of Swiss cheese in each pocket. Toothpicks are used to close the bag.

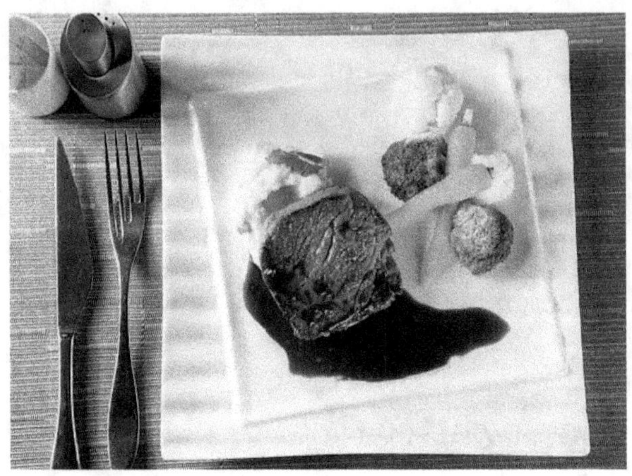

4. Combine the flour, garlic powder, paprika, salt, and pepper in a shallow dish.

5. Beat the eggs in a separate shallow bowl.

6. Combine the breadcrumbs and a sprinkle of salt in a third shallow dish.

7. Cover each chicken breast with the flour mixture, then the egg mixture, and lastly, the breadcrumbs.

8. In a large pan over medium-high heat, heat the vegetable oil. Cook until the chicken breasts are golden brown on both sides, approximately 5 minutes.

9. Place the chicken in a baking dish and bake for 20-25 minutes or until the internal temperature reaches 165°F.

10. Remove the toothpicks and serve immediately.

11. With a side salad or your favourite vegetable dish, serve your homemade Chicken Cordon Bleu.

8.2.4 Wellington of beef

Beef Wellington is a traditional and elegant meal ideal for a special occasion. Here's a recipe you can make at home:

Ingredients:

- 1 1/2 pounds tenderloin beef
- seasoned with salt & pepper
- 2 tbsp of olive oil
- 1 tablespoon Dijon mustard
- 1/4 cup fresh herbs, chopped (such as thyme, rosemary, and parsley)
- 2 tbsp. melted butter
- 2 cups mushrooms, finely chopped
- 1/4 cup shallots, chopped
- a quarter cup of red wine

* 1 sheet thawed frozen puff pastry
* 1 beaten egg
* 1 teaspoon milk

Instructions:

1. Preheat the oven to 425 degrees Fahrenheit.
2. Season the beef tenderloin with salt and pepper to taste.

3. In a large pan over high heat, heat the olive oil. Sear the beef on both sides until it is browned, approximately 2-3 minutes on each side. Set aside after removing from the skillet.

4. Combine the dijon mustard and chopped herbs in a small bowl. Spread the sauce all over the cooked meat.

5. Melt the butter in the same skillet over medium heat. Cook, stirring occasionally, until the mushrooms are soft and the liquid has evaporated, approximately 5-7 minutes. Cook for another 2-3 minutes, or until the liquid has reduced, before adding the red wine.

6. Roll out the puff pastry to approximately 1/4 inch thickness on a floured board. In the middle of the puff pastry, place the seared meat.

7. Serve the mushroom mixture on top of the meat.

8. Fold the puff pastry over the meat and mushroom mixture, tucking in the ends to make a tight package. Put the beef Wellington on a baking sheet lined with parchment paper, seam side down.

9. Mix the egg and milk in a small bowl to produce an egg wash. Brush the puff pastry with the egg wash.

10. Bake for 35-40 minutes until the puff pastry is golden brown and the beef reaches an internal temperature of 135°F for medium-rare or 145°F for medium.\

11. Let 10 minutes for the beef Wellington to rest before slicing and serving. Enjoy!

Quiche Lorraine is a traditional French cuisine that may be served for any occasion, from a formal breakfast to a casual supper at home. Here's how to create your own delectable Quiche Lorraine:

Ingredients:

- 1 pie crust (pre-made)
- 6 eggs
- 1-quart thick cream
- 1-quart milk

- 1 teaspoon of salt
- 1/4 teaspoon ground black pepper
- a quarter teaspoon of nutmeg
- 6 cooked and crumbled bacon slices
- 1 cup Swiss cheese, shredded

Instructions:

1. Preheat the oven to 375 degrees Fahrenheit (190 degrees Celsius).

2. Lay out the pie dough and line a 9-inch pie plate with it. Set aside after crimping the edges.

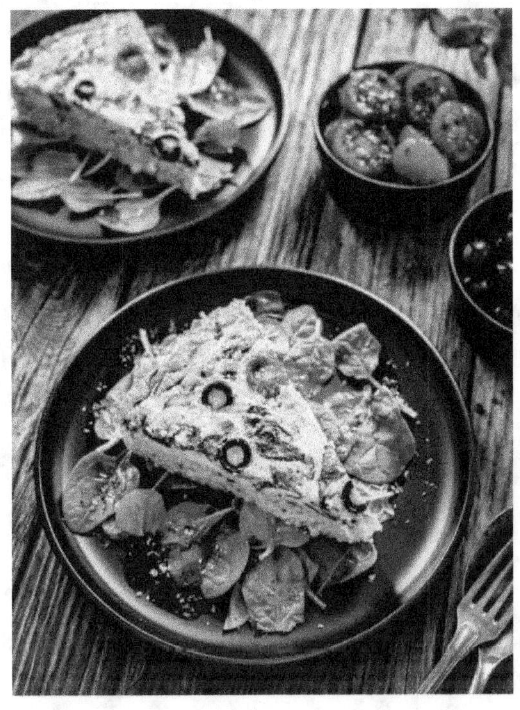

3. Add the eggs, heavy cream, milk, salt, pepper, and nutmeg in a medium mixing bowl.

4. Scatter the cooked and broken bacon on the bottom of the pie crust. Top with shredded Swiss cheese.

5. Over the bacon and cheese, pour the egg mixture.

6. Bake for 40-45 minutes, until the filling, is set and the top is golden brown, in a preheated oven.

7. Let 10-15 minutes for the Quiche Lorraine to cool before slicing and serving.

8. Enjoy your tasty Quiche, Lorraine!

8.2.5 Tiramisu (tiramisu)

Tiramisu is a traditional Italian dessert that is popular all over the globe. It's produced by stacking ladyfingers soaked in espresso and liquor with a thick mascarpone cheese and egg combination, then sprinkling with cocoa powder. Here is a recipe for homemade tiramisu:

Ingredients:

- 6 egg whites
- 3/4 cup granulated sugar
- 1 cup milk
- 1-quart thick cream
- a half teaspoon of vanilla extract
- 1 pound of mascarpone
- 1/4 cup freshly made espresso
- 14 cups of booze (such as Marsala, Amaretto, or Kahlua)
- Ladyfingers 24
- Dusting cocoa powder

Instructions:

1. Mix the egg yolks and sugar in a medium saucepan until thoroughly mixed.

2. Place the pot over medium heat and whisk in the milk. Heat, frequently whisking, for 8-10 minutes or until the mixture thickens and coats the back of a spoon.

3. Take the pan from the heat and set it aside to cool to room temperature.

4. Whip the heavy cream and vanilla extract in a large mixing bowl until soft peaks form.

5. Mascarpone cheese, in a separate bowl, whisks until smooth.

6. Stir the mascarpone cheese into the chilled egg mixture until thoroughly mixed.

7. Combine the espresso and liquor in a small dish.

8. Dip each ladyfinger in the espresso mixture, rotating to cover both sides and arranging in a single layer in a 9x13-inch dish.

9. Half of the mascarpone mixture should be spread over the ladyfingers.

10. Repeat with the remaining mascarpone mixture and soaked ladyfingers.

11. Refrigerate for at least 2 hours, preferably overnight, after wrapping the dish in plastic wrap.

12. Dust the top of the tiramisu with cocoa powder before serving.

13. Enjoy this luscious and decadent dessert!

9.0 Beverages and Smoothies

9.1 Pregnancy-friendly beverages and smoothies

Eating healthy meals and beverages throughout pregnancy is essential to promote the health and development of the developing baby. Smoothies and nutritious beverages may be a terrific way to get critical vitamins, minerals, and nutrients conveniently and enjoyably. Here are some pregnancy-friendly nutritional beverages and smoothies:

Green smoothie: This smoothie is loaded with vitamin and mineral-rich leafy greens. Combine spinach, kale, banana, almond milk, and a scoop of protein powder for a nutritious and satisfying drink.
Berries are abundant in antioxidants, which may help protect cells from harm. Combine strawberries, blueberries, and raspberries with Greek yoghurt and honey for a pleasant and healthy drink.

Ginger tea: Ginger has anti-inflammatory effects and helps alleviate morning sickness. For a calming and nourishing drink, steep grated ginger in hot water for a few minutes before adding honey and lemon.
Turmeric latte: Turmeric is an anti-inflammatory that may aid digestion. Combine turmeric powder, coconut milk,

honey, and cinnamon to make a warming and nourishing drink.

Beetroot juice is strong in folate, which is essential for embryonic development. Combine beets, apple, ginger, and lemon juice for a delicious and healthy drink.

Chia seed smoothie: Chia seeds have a high concentration of omega-3 fatty acids essential for brain development. Combine chia seeds, almond milk, banana, and honey for a satisfying and healthy drink.

Avocado smoothies are abundant in healthy fats and folate, both essential for embryonic growth. Combine avocado, almond milk, spinach, and honey for a creamy and healthy drink.

Carrot juice contains beta-carotene, which is essential for prenatal development. Combine carrots, apple, ginger, and lemon juice for a delicious and healthful drink.

Almond milk latte: Almond milk has a lot of calcium, which is good for prenatal bone growth. Combine almond milk, espresso, and honey to make a delightful and healthful drink.

Although these beverages and smoothies are healthful, they should be drunk in moderation since they may include extra sweets and calories. Consultation with a healthcare physician or trained dietitian may also assist you in fulfilling your particular dietary requirements throughout pregnancy.

Here's a healthy green smoothie recipe:

Ingredients:

- 2 cups spinach leaves, fresh
- 1 banana, ripe
- 1 cup pineapple chunks, frozen
- a half-cup almond milk
- 1/2 cup plain Greek yoghurt
- 1 tablespoon honey

Instructions:

1. Rinse and place the spinach leaves in a blender.

2. Combine the banana, frozen pineapple pieces, almond milk, Greek yoghurt, and honey in a blender.
3. Mix all of the ingredients until the smoothie is creamy and smooth.

4. Pour the green smoothie into a glass and serve immediately.

The spinach and pineapple in this green smoothie are high in nutrients and antioxidants. The banana gives natural sweetness, while the Greek yoghurt contains protein and calcium. The almond milk adds creaminess and a nutty taste to the smoothie. Enjoy this tasty and healthful smoothie as a snack or breakfast throughout your pregnancy.

Here's a tasty and healthy berry smoothie recipe that's ideal for pregnancy:

Ingredients:

- 1 cup berries, mixed (fresh or frozen)
- one banana
- 1/2 cup Greek yoghurt, plain
- half-cup almond milk (or milk of choice)
- 1 teaspoon honey (optional)
- a half teaspoon of vanilla extract
- 1 cup cubed ice

Instructions:

1. In a blender, combine all of the ingredients.

2. Mix until the mixture is smooth and creamy.

3. Add extra almond milk if the smoothie is too thick.

4. Pour into a glass and serve right away.

This smoothie is high in antioxidants from the mixed berries and vitamin C from the banana, making it an excellent option for supporting your immune system while pregnant. Greek yoghurt has protein and calcium, while almond milk contains healthy fats and additional calcium. Honey and vanilla essence provide natural sweetness without the need for extra sugar. Serve as a light breakfast or snack.

9.2.3 Ginger tea

Here's how to make ginger tea:

Ingredients:

- 1 inch peeled and grated fresh ginger root
- 2 cups of water
- 1 teaspoon honey (optional)
- 1 lemon (juiced) (optional)

Instructions:

1. Bring the water to a boil in a small saucepan.

2. Simmer for 10 minutes after adding the grated ginger root to the saucepan.

3. She rubbed the ginger tea from the heat through a fine mesh strainer.

4. If desired, season with honey and lemon juice.

5. Serve immediately and enjoy.

Ginger tea is an excellent choice for pregnant women since it may help relieve nausea and vomiting, both prevalent throughout pregnancy. It has anti-inflammatory qualities and may help enhance the immune system.

9.2.4 Turmeric powder

Here's how to make Turmeric Latte:

Ingredients:

- 1 cup almond milk, unsweetened
- 1 teaspoon turmeric powder
- 1 tablespoon honey or maple syrup
- 1 teaspoon ground cinnamon
- 1 teaspoon ground ginger
- 1 tsp black pepper

Instructions:

1. Warm the almond milk in a small saucepan over medium heat until hot but not boiling.

2. Whisk in the turmeric, honey or maple syrup, cinnamon, ginger, and black pepper until thoroughly blended.

3. Lower the heat to low and stir the mixture for 5-7 minutes.

4. Pour the mixture into a cup and serve immediately once it has been cooked and the spices have been absorbed into the milk.

You may alter the sweetness and spice levels to your liking. You may also use other kinds of milk for almond milk, such as coconut or cashew milk.

9.2.5 Red beet juice

Here's how to make Beetroot Juice:

Ingredients:

- 2 medium-sized beets
- 1 apple
- one carrot
- 1 lemon
- 1-inch ginger slice

- Water

Instructions:

1. Peel and wash the beets, apples, and carrot.

2. Chop them into little pieces small enough to put in your juicer.

3. Peel and chop the ginger into smaller pieces.

4. Squeeze the lemon and set aside the juice.

5. Juice the beets, apple, carrot, and ginger in a juicer.
6. Incorporate the lemon juice into the juice.

7. If the juice is excessively thick, dilute it with water.

8. Chill before serving.

You may modify the juice's sweetness and sharpness by add6.ing more or less apple and lemon juice.

9.3 Refreshing and hydrating beverage recipes

Here are some ideas for hydrating and refreshing drinks:

1. Water with Cucumber and Lemon:

- One cucumber and 1 lemon, sliced, should be added to a big pitcher of water.
- Let it chill for a few hours to enable the flavours to meld.
- Pour over ice for a pleasant and hydrating beverage.

2. Cooler with Watermelon and Mint:
- Puree 4 cups cubed watermelon, 1/4 cup fresh mint leaves, and 1 tablespoon honey in a blender.
- Blend in the ice until smooth.
- Serve in a large glass garnished with a sprig of fresh mint.

3. Green Tea Iced with Honey and Lemon:
- Make 4 cups of green tea and set it aside to cool.
- Stir in 2 tablespoons of honey and the juice of 1 lemon until the honey is dissolved.
- Place the tea in the refrigerator to cool.
- Garnish with a lemon slice and serve over ice.

4. Coconut Pineapple Water:
- Combine 1 cup pineapple chunks and 2 cups coconut water in a blender.
- Blend in the ice until smooth.
- Serve in a large glass with a slice of pineapple for garnish.

5. Lassi de Mango:

- One cup diced ripe mango, 1 cup plain Greek yoghurt, 1/2 cup milk, and 1 tablespoon of honey in a blender.
- Blend in the ice until smooth.
- Serve in a large glass with a garnish of powdered cardamom.

10.0 Treating Pregnancy-Related Conditions

10.1 Nutritional guidelines for gestational diabetes,

preeclampsia, and other disorders

Gestational diabetes and preeclampsia are both frequent pregnancy complications. Good eating may help manage these issues and ensure a safe pregnancy.

Eating a nutritious diet is essential to control blood sugar levels during pregnancy. This involves eating frequent meals with a healthy mix of carbs, proteins, and fats. Whole grains, fruits, and vegetables with a low glycemic index are also advised. It is critical to avoid meals containing added sugars and processed carbs.

A low-sodium diet is often prescribed for preeclampsia to assist in regulating blood pressure. This entails reducing processed foods and avoiding salt in meals. Foods high in potassium, such as bananas, sweet potatoes, and avocados, may also help regulate blood pressure.
Some illnesses like anaemia or acid reflux may need dietary modifications. Iron-rich meals such as red meat, legumes, and leafy greens are advised for anaemia. Avoiding trigger foods like spicy or fatty foods and eating smaller, more often meals may assist with acid reflux.

Speaking with a healthcare expert is critical for tailored dietary advice based on individual requirements and situations.

Pregnancy is crucial for women to focus on their health and food to ensure their bodies have all the nutrients they need to support the developing baby. Nevertheless, some women may develop pregnancy-related disorders such as gestational diabetes, preeclampsia, and morning sickness, which may need dietary changes. Here are some recipe suggestions for these conditions:

1. **Diabetes during pregnancy:**

Diabetes that develops during pregnancy is known as gestational diabetes. Women with this illness must control their blood sugar levels by eating a well-balanced diet rich in complex carbs, lean protein, and healthy fats. Here are some recipes for gestational diabetes:

- Grilled chicken with quinoa and roasted veggies
- Salmon baked in the oven with steamed broccoli and brown rice Chilli with turkey, kidney beans, and mixed veggies

Greek yoghurt topped with berries and almonds
Preeclampsia:

Preeclampsia is a pregnancy-related illness marked by high blood pressure and organ damage, particularly to the liver and kidneys. Women with preeclampsia should eat a low-sodium diet to control their blood pressure. Some preeclampsia recipe ideas include:

- Chicken breast grilled with roasted veggies and sweet potatoes
- Steamed green beans and brown rice with grilled fish
- Salad with spinach, strawberries, almonds, and a low-sodium vinaigrette
- Greek yoghurt with sliced bananas and cinnamon sprinkled on top

Early morning sickness:

Morning sickness causes nausea and vomiting and is a frequent pregnancy-related symptom. Ladies suffering from morning sickness may find eating and keeping food down difficult. Here are some recipes for morning sickness:

- Lemon and honey ginger tea
- Hummus crackers with chopped veggies
- Smoothies made with Greek yoghurt, berries, and greens
- Soups made with broth, veggies, and lean protein

These recipes are not intended to replace medical advice, and pregnant women should always contact their healthcare professionals for customized nutritional recommendations.